Elsevier's Integrated

Immunology
and Microbiology

Elsevier's Integrated
Immunology
and Microbiology

Jeffrey K. Actor PhD

Associate Professor
Department of Pathology and Laboratory Medicine
University of Texas-Houston Medical School
Houston, Texas

1600 John F. Kennedy Blvd
Suite 1800
Philadelphia, PA 19103-2899

ELSEVIER'S INTEGRATED IMMUNOLOGY
AND MICROBIOLOGY

ISBN-13: 978-0-323-03389-3
ISBN-10: 0-323-03389-X

Notice

Knowledge and best practice in this field are constantly changing. As new research and experience broaden our knowledge, changes in practice, treatment and drug therapy may become necessary or appropriate. Readers are advised to check the most current information provided (i) on procedures featured or (ii) by the manufacturer of each product to be administered, to verify the recommended dose or formula, the method and duration of administration, and contraindications. It is the responsibility of the practitioner, relying on their own experience and knowledge of the patient, to make diagnoses, to determine dosages and the best treatment for each individual patient, and to take all appropriate safety precautions. To the fullest extent of the law, neither the Publisher nor the Author assumes any liability for any injury and/or damage to persons or property arising out or related to any use of the material contained in this book.

The Publisher

Library of Congress Cataloging-in-Publication Data

Actor, Jeffrey K.
    Elsevier's integrated immunology & microbiology / Jeffrey K. Actor.—1st ed.
        p.   ;   cm.
    ISBN 0-323-03389-X
    1. Immunology. 2. Microbiology. I. Title. II. Title: Elsevier's integrated immunology and microbiology. III. Title: Integrated immunology and microbiology.
    [DNLM: 1. Immunology. 2. Microbiology. QW 540 A188e 2007]
    QR181.A258 2007
    616.07'9—dc22

                                                                    2006048247

Acquisitions Editor: Alex Stibbe
Developmental Editor: Andrew Hall

Printed in China

Last digit is the print number: 9   8   7   6   5   4   3   2   1

To my father, Paul Actor, PhD, who instilled in me a sense of excitement about the wonders of science and the curiosity to ask questions about biological systems

Preface

Immunology represents a rapidly changing field, with new theories actively evolving as molecular techniques broaden our scientific perspective on interactions between pathogens and humans. The immune cells and organs of the body comprise the primary defense system against invasion by microorganisms. A functional immune system confers a state of health through effective immune surveillance and elimination of infectious agents. The study of immunologic and hematologic principles, as applied toward understanding host protection against pathogenic assault, integrates well with microbiology and the study of basic concepts underlying the nature of foreign pathogens. The goal of the first half of the book is to present immune system components, both innate and adaptive, in a concise manner to elucidate their intertwined relationships that culminate in effective host protection and health. The remaining chapters present the world of microbiology, with a concise overview of clinically relevant bacteria, viruses, fungi, and parasites, to allow an understanding of infectious organisms as the causative agents underlying human disease.

This book is aimed toward students of human health and those within the medical profession; it is written to simplify concepts and encourage the inquisitive individual to explore further medically relevant topics. Indeed, the purpose of the integrated text series is to encourage cross-disciplinary thought across multiple sciences. Integration boxes promote cross-discipline thinking, and allow the reader to build bridges between related concepts in other medical fields. The clinical vignettes and associated questions at the back of the book are organized to provide perspectives into molecular aspects underlying clinical disease manifestation. These scenarios are aimed to assist in understanding consequences of ineffective, inappropriate, overactive, or nonregulated responses and their relationship to immunologic disorders and deficiencies, as well as to responses occurring during infection.

Overall the text attempts to present information in a clinically relevant and concise manner that outlines concepts for further exploration, creating a base of knowledge for those with a desire to understand how the healthy individual combats disease.

Jeffrey K. Actor, PhD

Editorial Review Board

Acknowledgments

I would like to thank Robert L. Hunter, Jr., MD, Ph.D., and Steven J. Norris, Ph.D., who supported and encouraged me as I strove to reach my academic and research goals. A special thanks goes to Alexandra Stibbe at Elsevier for her vision and insights that made the *Integrated Series* possible and to Andrew C. Hall for his attention to detail, his humor, and his positive guidance.

Contents

Series Preface

How to Use This Book

The idea for Elsevier's Integrated Series came about at a seminar on the USMLE Step 1 exam at an American Medical Student Association (AMSA) meeting. We noticed that the discussion between faculty and students focused on how the exams were becoming increasingly integrated—with case scenarios and questions often combining two or three science disciplines. The students were clearly concerned about how they could best integrate their basic science knowledge.

One faculty member gave some interesting advice: "read through your textbook in, say, biochemistry, and every time you come across a section that mentions a concept or piece of information relating to another basic science—for example, immunology—highlight that section in the book. Then go to your immunology textbook and look up this information, and make sure you have a good understanding of it. When you have, go back to your biochemistry textbook and carry on reading."

This was a great suggestion—if only students had the time, and all of the books necessary at hand, to do it! At Elsevier we thought long and hard about a way of simplifying this process, and eventually the idea for Elsevier's Integrated Series was born.

The series centers on the concept of the *integration box*. These boxes occur throughout the text whenever a link to another basic science is relevant. They're easy to spot in the text—with their color-coded headings and logos. Each box contains a title for the integration topic and then a brief summary of the topic. The information is complete in itself—you probably won't have to go to any other sources—and you have the basic knowledge to use as a foundation if you want to expand your knowledge of the topic.

You can use this book in two ways. First, as a review book . . .
When you are using the book for review, the integration boxes will jog your memory on topics you have already covered. You'll be able to reassure yourself that you can identify the link, and you can quickly compare your knowledge of the topic with the summary in the box. The integration boxes might highlight gaps in your knowledge, and then you can use them to determine what topics you need to cover in more detail.

Second, the book can be used as a short text to have at hand while you are taking your course . . .
You may come across an integration box that deals with a topic you haven't covered yet, and this will ensure that you're one step ahead in identifying the links to other subjects (especially useful if you're working on a PBL exercise). On a simpler level, the links in the boxes to other sciences and to clinical medicine will help you see clearly the relevance of the basic science topic you are studying. You may already be confident in the subject matter of many of the integration boxes, so they will serve as helpful reminders.

At the back of the book we have included case study questions relating to each chapter so that you can test yourself as you work your way through the book.

Online Version

An online version of the book is available on our Student Consult site. Use of this site is free to anyone who has bought the printed book. Please see the inside front cover for full details on the Student Consult and how to access the electronic version of this book.

In addition to containing USMLE test questions, fully searchable text, and an image bank, the Student Consult site offers additional integration links, both to the other books in Elsevier's Integrated Series and to other key Elsevier textbooks.

Books in Elsevier's Integrated Series

The nine books in the series cover all of the basic sciences. The more books you buy in the series, the more links are made accessible across the series, both in print and online.

 Anatomy and Embryology

 Histology

 Neuroscience

 Biochemistry

 Physiology

 Pathology

 Immunology and Microbiology

 Pharmacology

 Genetics

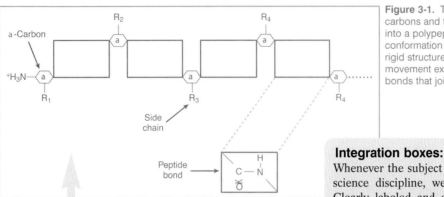

Figure 3-1. The peptide bond linking α-carbons and their side chains together into a polypeptide. The *trans* conformation is favored, producing a rigid structure that restricts freedom of movement except for rotation around bonds that join to the α-carbons.

Integration boxes:
Whenever the subject matter can be related to another science discipline, we've put in an Integration Box. Clearly labeled and color-coded, these boxes include nuggets of information on topics that require an integrated knowledge of the sciences to be fully understood. The material in these boxes is complete in itself, and you can use them as a way of reminding yourself of information you already know and reinforcing key links between the sciences. Or the boxes may contain information you have not come across before, in which case you can use them a springboard for further research or simply to appreciate the relevance of the subject matter of the book to the study of medicine.

Artwork:
The books are packed with 4-color illustrations and photographs. When a concept can be better explained with a picture, we've drawn one. Where possible, the pictures tell a dynamic story that will help you remember the information far more effectively than a paragraph of text.

MICROBIOLOGY

Prion Diseases

Prions (PrP^{Sc}) are formed from otherwise normal neurologic proteins (PrP) and are responsible for encephalopathies in humans (Creutzfeldt-Jakob disease, kuru), scrapie in sheep, and bovine spongiform encephalopathy. Contact between the normal PrP and PrP^{Sc} results in conversion of the secondary structure of PrP from predominantly α-helical to predominantly β-pleated sheet. The altered structure of the protein forms long, filamentous aggregates that gradually damage neuronal tissue. The harmful PrP^{Sc} form is highly resistant to heat, UV irradiation, and protease enzymes.

Figure 3-3. Secondary structure includes α-helix and β-pleated sheet (β-sheet).

Since proline has no free hydrogen to contribute to helix stability, it is referred to as a "helix breaker." The α-helix is found in most globular proteins and in some fibrous proteins (e.g., α-keratin).

Text:
Succinct, clearly written text, focusing on the core information you need to know and no more. It's the same level as a carefully prepared course syllabus or lecture notes.

rmation

-structure) consists of

tabilized by hydrogen

f adjacent sequences.

(parallel) or opposite (antiparallel) direction. β-Structures are found in 80% of all globular proteins and in silk fibroin.

Supersecondary Structure and Domains

Supersecondary structures, or *motifs*, are characteristic combinations of secondary structure 10–40 residues in length that recur in different proteins. They bridge the gap between the less specific regularity of secondary structure and the highly specific folding of tertiary structure. The same motif can perform similar functions in different proteins.

- The four-helix bundle motif provides a cavity for enzymes to bind prosthetic groups or cofactors.
- The β-barrel motif can bind hydrophobic molecules such as retinol in the interior of the barrel.
- Motifs may also be mixtures of both α and β conformations.

Immunology

Introduction to Immunity and Immune Systems

1

●●● CHIEF FUNCTION OF IMMUNITY

The immune cells and organs of the body make up the primary defense system against invasion by microorganisms and foreign pathogens. A functional immune system confers a state of health through effective elimination of infectious agents (bacteria, viruses, fungi, and parasites) and through control of malignancies by protective immune surveillance. In essence, the process is based in functional discernment between self and non-self, a process that begins in utero and continues through adult life.

Immune responses are designed to interact with the environment to protect the host against pathogenic invaders. The goal of the chapters in Section I is to appreciate the components of the human immune response that work together to protect the host. In addition, a working clinical understanding of the concept of immune-based diseases resulting from either immune system component deficiencies or excess activity will be presented.

●●● INNATE IMMUNE SYSTEM

The immune system consists of two overlapping compartments representing interactions between innate and adaptive components and associated responses. The innate immune mechanisms provide the first line of defense from infectious disease (Table 1-1). Innate immune components are present from birth and consist of nonspecific components available prior to the onset of infection. Innate immune recognition utilizes preformed effector molecules to recognize broad structural motifs that are highly conserved within microbial species. Engagement of innate components leads to triggering of signal pathways to promote inflammation, ensuring that invading pathogens remain in check while the specific immune response is either generated or up-regulated.

●●● ADAPTIVE IMMUNE SYSTEM

The adaptive (also called "acquired") immune response accounts for specificity in recognition of foreign substances, or antigens, by functional receptors residing on the surface of B and T lymphocytes (Table 1-2 and Fig. 1-1). The B-cell antigen receptor (BCR) is the surface immunoglobulin, an integral glycosylated membrane protein with unique regions that bind specific antigens. There can be thousands of identical copies present on the surface of a single cell. B-cell activation occurs upon interaction of the BCR with antigen, leading to cell activation and differentiation into plasma cells, which secrete soluble immunoglobulins, or antibodies. B cells and antibodies together make up the humoral immune response. The T cell has a surface receptor structurally similar to the antibody, which also recognizes specific antigenic determinants (*epitopes*). T cells control the cellular arm of the immune response. Unlike the antibody, the T-cell receptor is present only on its surface and is not secreted. The process of T-cell activation requires a third group of cells called *antigen-presenting cells* (APCs). APCs contain surface molecules,

---

BIOCHEMISTRY

Mediators of Acute Inflammation

Metabolism of phospholipids is required for production of prostaglandins and leukotrienes, both of which enhance inflammatory response by promoting increased vascular permeability and vasodilation. Prostaglandins are 20-carbon fatty acid derivatives containing a cyclopentane ring and an oxygen-containing functional group; leukotrienes are 20-carbon fatty acid derivatives containing three conjugated double bonds and hydroxyl groups.

TABLE 1-1. Innate Defensive Components

Component	Effectors	Function
Anatomic and physiologic barriers	Skin and mucous membranes Temperature, acidic pH, lactic acid Chemical mediators	Physical barriers to limit entry, spread, and replication of pathogens
Inflammatory mediators	Complement Cytokines and interferons Lysozymes Acute-phase proteins and lactoferrin Leukotrienes and prostaglandins	Direct lysis of pathogen or infected cells Activation of other immune components Bacterial cell wall destruction Mediation of response Vasodilation and increased vascular permeability
Cellular components	Polymorphonuclear cells • Neutrophils, eosinophils • Basophils, mast cells Phagocytic-endocytic cells • Monocytes and macrophages • Dendritic cells	Phagocytosis and intracellular destruction of microorganisms Presentation of foreign antigen to lymphocytes

TABLE 1-2. Key Elements of the Innate and Adaptive Immune Systems

Innate	Adaptive (Acquired)
Rapid response (minutes to hours)	Slow response (days to weeks)
PMNs and phagocytes	B cells and T cells
Preformed effectors with limited variability Pattern recognition molecules recognizing structural motifs	B-cell and T-cell receptors with a diverse array of highly selective specificities
Soluble activators	Antibodies (humoral response)
Proinflammatory mediators	Cytokines (cellular response)
Nonspecific	Specific
No memory, no increase in response upon secondary exposure	Memory, maturation of secondary response

PMNs, polymorphonuclear neutrophils.

human leukocyte antigens (HLAs), which are encoded within a gene region known as the major histocompatibility complex (MHC). Together these groups of molecules form a regulated pathway to present foreign antigens for subsequent recognition and triggering of specific responses to protect against disease.

●●● SPECIFICITY OF ADAPTIVE RESPONSE BY LYMPHOCYTE RECEPTORS

Each B and T lymphocyte expresses a unique antigen receptor. The generation of antigen-binding specificity occurs prior to antigen exposure through a DNA rearrangement process that creates receptors of high diversity and binding potential. During an active immune response, a small number of B- and T-cell clones bind to the antigen with high affinity and then undergo activation, proliferation, and differentiation (Fig. 1-2). This process is called clonal selection and leads to both the production of multiple cells all with the same antigen recognition capability and to the generation of immunologic memory.

Long-term good health requires continued discrimination against foreign agents dependent upon immunologic memory in which the adaptive immune system can more efficiently respond to previously encountered antigens (Fig. 1-3). The specific adaptive response against an antigen is much greater during secondary exposure. This principle accounts for the clinical utility of vaccines, which have done more to improve mortality rates worldwide than any other medical discovery in recorded history.

●●● TIGHT REGULATION OF THE IMMUNE SYSTEM AND ASSOCIATED RESPONSES

Immunologic diseases can be grouped into two large categories: deficiency and dysfunction (Fig. 1-4). Immunodeficiency diseases occur as the result of the absence of one or more elements of the immune system; this can either be congenital or acquired after birth. Immune dysfunction occurs when a particular immune response develops that is detrimental to the host. This deleterious response may be against a foreign or a self-antigen. It may also be an inappropriate regulation of an effector response that serves to prevent a protective response. Notwithstanding, the host is adversely affected. A healthy immune system occurs as a result of balance between innate and adaptive immunity, cellular and humoral immunity (see Chapters 3 and 4), inflammatory and regulatory networks

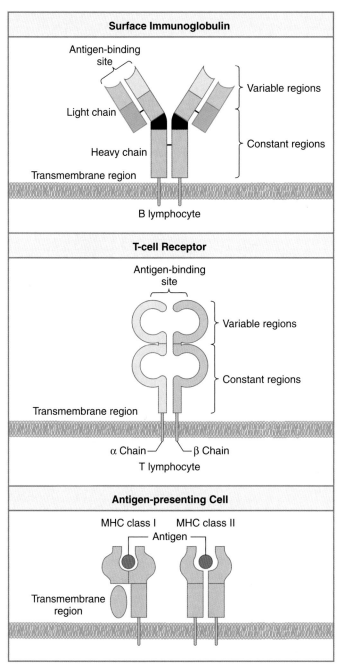

Figure 1-1. Basic structure of antigen receptors on the surface of a B cell (the immunoglobulin B-cell receptor, BCR), a T-cell (the T-cell receptor, TCR), and major histocompatibility complex (MHC) molecules.

(see Chapter 6), and small biochemical mediators (cytokines) (see Chapter 7). Disease occurs when the balance is altered by either deficiency or dysfunction.

KEY POINTS ABOUT IMMUNOLOGY AND THE IMMUNE SYSTEM

- The chief function of the immune system is to distinguish between self and non-self.

- The immune system consists of two overlapping compartments: the innate immune system and the adaptive immune system.

- The specificity of the adaptive immune system is due to antigen-specific receptors (immunoglobulins and T-cell receptors). The generation of antigen-binding diversity inherent in these receptors occurs prior to antigen exposure through DNA rearrangement.

- To generate an active immune response against a certain antigen, a small number of B- and T-cell clones that bind to the antigen with high affinity undergo activation, proliferation, and differentiation into plasma cells (for B cells) or activated T cells. This process is called clonal selection.

- The adaptive immune system has memory, meaning that the response against a foreign substance is much greater after the first exposure.

- Furthermore, the immune system is tightly regulated to ensure appropriate activation.

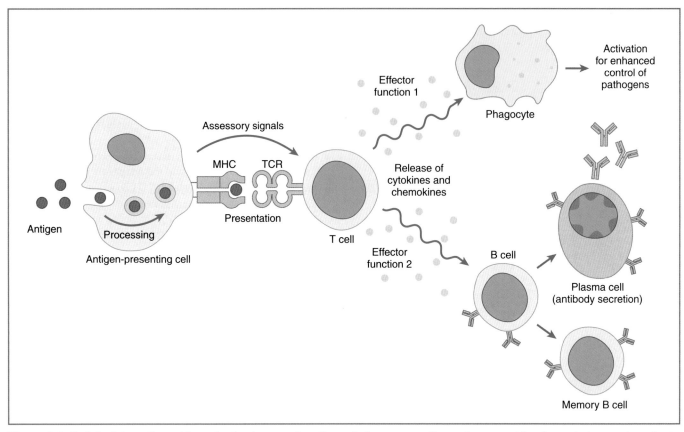

Figure 1-2. Cellular interactions drive adaptive immune functions. Antigen-presenting cells present foreign substances to activate T cells. T cells differentiate to become effectors to help phagocytes control pathogen infection or to assist B cells in production and secretion of immunoglobulins.

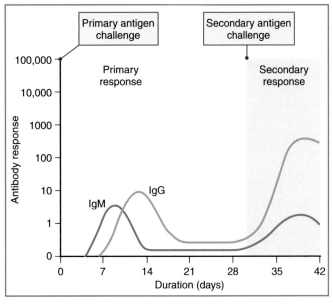

Figure 1-3. Primary and secondary antibody responses. The adaptive immune system has memory, allowing for maturation of a rapid secondary immune response with higher specificity and magnitude directed against foreign substances.

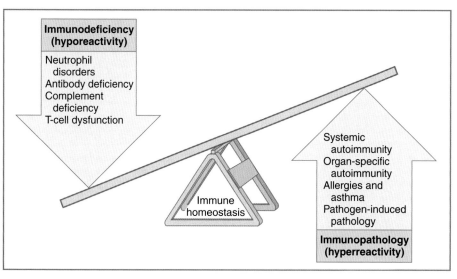

Figure 1-4. Immunodeficiency and dysfunction. Immune-based diseases can be caused by lack of specific functions (immunodeficiency) or by excessive activity (hypersensitivity).

Cells and Organs of the Immune System   2

The first line of defense against infection includes natural physical barriers that limit entry of microorganisms into the body. The skin, mucosal epithelia, and cilia lining the respiratory tract represent effective mechanical barriers. Biochemical mechanisms also support innate processes to ward off potential pathogens, including sebaceous gland secretions that contain fatty acids, hydrolytic enzymes, and antibacterial defensins. Enzymes in saliva and intestinal secretions that are capable of digesting bacterial cell walls and the acidic pH of the stomach lumen all represent innate barriers to infection. Once a pathogen has compromised these barriers and gained access to the body, cellular components must be evoked to combat invading organisms.

●●● PLURIPOTENT HEMATOPOIETIC STEM CELLS

Immune system cells are derived from pluripotent hematopoietic stem cells in the bone marrow. These cells are functionally grouped into two major categories of immune response: *innate* (natural) and *acquired* (adaptive). Innate immunity is present from birth and consists of nonspecific components. Acquired immunity by definition requires recognition specificity to foreign (*non-self*) substances (*antigens*). The major properties of the acquired immune response are specificity, memory, adaptiveness, and discrimination between self and non-self.

The acquired immune response is further classified as *humoral* or *cellular* immunity, based on participation of two major cell types. Humoral immunity involves B lymphocytes that synthesize and secrete antibodies to neutralize pathogens and toxins. Cell-mediated immunity (CMI) involves effector T lymphocytes, which can lyse infected target cells or secrete immunoregulatory factors following interaction with antigen-presenting cells (APCs) to combat intracellular viruses and organisms.

An intricate communication system allows components of innate and acquired immunity to work in concert to combat infectious disease. *Leukocytes* provide either innate or specific adaptive immunity and are derived from *myeloid* or *lymphoid* lineage (Fig. 2-1). The production of leukocytes is induced by hematopoietic growth factor glycoproteins that exert critical regulatory functions in the processes of proliferation, differentiation, and functional activation of hematopoietic progenitors and mature blood cells. Myeloid cells include highly phagocytic, motile polymorphonuclear neutrophils, monocytes, and macrophages (tissue resident monocytes) that provide a first line of defense against most pathogens. The other myeloid cells, including polymorphonuclear

HISTOLOGY

Pluripotent Hemopoietic Stem Cells

Pluripotent hemopoietic stem cells differentiate into myeloid and lymphoid lineages. The myeloid lineage gives rise to histologically distinct neutrophils with a characteristic multilobed nucleus, basophils with azurophilic granules and S-shaped nucleus, and eosinophils with red-orange specific granules and a bilobed nucleus, as well as to erythrocytes, monocytes, and platelets. Lymphoid lineages give rise to B and T lymphocytes.

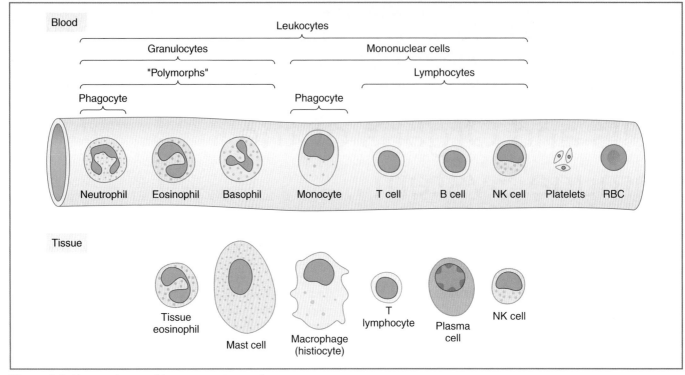

Figure 2-1. Nomenclature of immune system cells.

eosinophils, basophils, and their tissue counterparts—mast cells—are involved in defense against parasites and in the genesis of allergic reactions. Cells from the lymphoid lineage are responsible for humoral (B lymphocytes) and cell-mediated (T lymphocytes) immunity (Table 2-1).

●●● MYELOID CELLS: FIRST LINE OF DEFENSE

Neutrophils

Granulocyte neutrophils are the most highly abundant myeloid cell type, comprising 40% to 70% of total white blood cells (WBCs). They are motile phagocytic leukocytes that are the first cells recruited to acute inflammatory sites. Neutrophils are short-lived and are produced within the bone marrow through stimulation with granulocyte–colony stimulating factor (G-CSF). They ingest, kill, and digest microbial pathogens, with their functions dependent upon special proteins found in primary granules (containing cationic defensins and myeloperoxidase) and secondary granules (iron chelators and digestive enzymes). Neutrophilic granules contain multiple antimicrobial agents including oxygen-independent lysozyme (peptidoglycan degradation) and lactoferrin (iron chelator). In addition, respiratory burst and granule oxidases can reduce molecular oxygen to superoxide radicals and reactive oxygen species to produce toxic metabolites (hydrogen peroxide) that limit bacterial growth. Neutrophils dying at the site of infection contribute to the formation of white pustules called *pus*.

Eosinophils

Eosinophils are polymorphonuclear granulocytes that defend against parasites and participate in hypersensitivity reactions via antibody-dependent cell-mediated cytotoxicity (ADCC) mechanisms. Their cytotoxicity is mediated by large cytoplasmic granules, which contain eosinophilic basic and cationic proteins. Eosinophils are involved in manifestation of allergy and asthma, via IgE-mediated antigen specificity.

Basophils and Mast Cells

Basophils and their tissue counterpart, mast cells, are polymorphonuclear granulocytes that produce cytokines in defense against parasites. These cells are also responsible for allergic inflammation. Basophils and mast cells display high-affinity surface membrane receptors for IgE antibodies. These cells degranulate when cell-bound IgE antibodies are cross-linked by antigens, secreting low-molecular-weight mediators that regulate vascular tone and capillary permeability from both primary (histamine, serotonin, and platelet-activating factor) and secondary granules (leukotrienes C_4, D_4, and B_4; prostaglandin D_2; and bradykinin). Mast cells arise from independent myeloid progenitor cells and also regulate IgE-mediated hypersensitivity responses.

Monocytes and Macrophages

Monocytes and macrophages are involved in phagocytosis and intracellular killing of microorganisms. Monocytes comprise up to 10% of circulating WBCs. Macrophages are

TABLE 2-1. Myeloid Leukocytes and Their Properties

Phenotype	Morphology	Circulating Differential Count*	Effector Function
Neutrophil	PMN granulocyte	2–7.5 × 10⁹/L	Phagocytosis and digestion of microbes
Eosinophil	PMN granulocyte	0.04–0.44 × 10⁹/L	Immediate hypersensitivity (allergic) reactions, defense against helminths
Basophil	PMN granulocyte	0–0.1 × 10⁹/L	Immediate hypersensitivity (allergic) reactions
Mast cell	PMN granulocyte	Tissue specific	Immediate hypersensitivity (allergic) reactions
Monocytes	Monocytic	0.2–0.8 × 10⁹/L	Circulating macrophage precursor
Macrophage	Monocytic	Tissue specific	Phagocytosis and digestion of microbes, antigen presentation to T cells
Dendritic cell	Monocytic	Tissue specific	Antigen presentation to naïve T cells, initiation of adaptive responses

PMN, polymorphonuclear.
*Normal range for 95% of population, +/– 2 standard deviations.

BIOCHEMISTRY

Vasoactive Mediators

A hallmark of inflammation includes the four cardinal signs of *tumor* (swelling), *rubor* (redness), *calor* (heat), and *dolor* (pain), resulting from biochemical actions of the vasoactive mediators prostaglandins and leukotrienes, produced from arachidonic acid precursors, and bradykinin, a peptide of the kinin group of proteins formed in response to activation of factor XII (Hageman factor). In general, these potent vasodilators cause contraction of nonvascular smooth muscle, increased vascular permeability, and pain.

terminally differentiated, long-lived monocytes residing in reticular connective tissue that comprises the *reticulo-endothelial system* (RES; also referred to as the *mononuclear phagocytic system* or *lymphoreticular system*). Monocytes and macrophages are motile, yet become highly adherent upon phagocytic activity; they provide natural immunity against microorganisms by a coupled process of phagocytosis and intracellular killing, recruiting other inflammatory cells through the production of cytokines and chemokines, and presenting peptide antigens to T lymphocytes for the production of antigen-specific immunity. The cells of the RES include circulating monocytes as well as tissue-resident macrophages in the spleen, lymph nodes, thymus, submucosal tissues of the respiratory and alimentary tracts, bone marrow, and connective tissues. Specialized macrophages include Kupffer cells in the liver, Langerhans cells in skin, and glial cells in the central nervous system.

Dendritic Cells

Dendritic cells are differentiated macrophages that act as APCs to activate helper T cells and cytotoxic cells (CTL) as well as B cells. They are found in epithelia and in most organs and are important initiators for adaptive immune recognition of foreign (non-self) proteins.

Platelets and Erythrocytes

Platelets and erythrocytes (red blood cells, RBCs) arise from myeloid megakaryocyte precursors. Platelets and erythrocytes are involved in blood clotting and release inflammatory mediators involved in innate immune activation.

●●● LYMPHOID CELLS: SPECIFIC AND LONG-LASTING IMMUNITY

Lymphoid cells are present in healthy adults at concentrations of approximately 1.3–3.5 × 10⁹/L. Lymphocytes differentiate into three separate lines: (1) thymic-dependent cells or T lymphocytes that operate in cellular and humoral immunity, (2) B lymphocytes that differentiate into plasma cells to secrete antibodies, and (3) natural killer (NK) cells that can lyse infected target cells. T and B lymphocytes produce and express specific receptors for antigens whereas natural killer (NK) cells do not (Table 2-2).

B Lymphocytes

B lymphocytes differentiate into *plasma cells* to secrete antibodies, which are immunoglobulin (Ig) glycoproteins that bind antigens with a high degree of specificity. The genesis of mature B cells from pluripotent progenitor stem cells occurs in the bone marrow and is antigen-independent. The activation of B cells into antibody-producing and -secreting cells (plasma cells) is antigen-dependent. Mature B cells can have 1–1.5 × 10⁵ immunoglobulin receptors for antigen (all of which have the same antigenic specificity) embedded within their plasma membrane. Once specific antigen binds to surface Ig molecule, the B cells differentiate into plasma cells that produce and secrete these antibodies. If B cells also

TABLE 2-2. Lymphoid Leukocytes and Their Properties

Total Lymphocytes	1.3–3.5 × 10⁹/L		Effector Function
B cell	Monocytic	Adaptive	Humoral immunity
Plasma cell	Monocytic	Adaptive	Terminally differentiated, antibody secreting B cell
T cell	Monocytic	Adaptive	Cell-mediated immunity
Natural killer cell	Monocytic	Innate	Innate response to microbial or viral infection

interact with T helper cells, they proliferate and switch the isotype (class) of immunoglobulin that is produced, while retaining the same antigen-binding specificity. T helper cells are thought to be required for switching from IgM to IgG, IgA, or IgE isotypes. B cells also process and present protein antigens. In this case, immunoglobulin receptors recognize and internalize antigen, which then is degraded and presented to T lymphocytes.

T Lymphocytes

Immature thymocytes differentiate in the thymus, where rearrangement of antigen-specific T-cell receptor (TCR) genes gives rise to a diverse set of clonotypic T lymphocytes. In the thymus, cells are selected for maturation only if their TCRs do not interact with self-peptides presented in the context of self–major histocompatibility complex (MHC) molecules on antigen-presenting cells. T lymphocytes are involved in the regulation of the immune response and in cell-mediated immunity, and help B cells produce antibody. Mature lymphocytes also display one of two accessory molecules—CD4 or CD8—which define whether a T cell will be a CD4-expressing *helper T lymphocyte* or a CD8-expressing *cytotoxic T lymphocyte* (CTL). Every T lymphocyte also expresses CD3, a multi-subunit cell-signaling complex noncovalently associated with the antigen-specific TCR. The TCR/CD3 complex recognizes antigens associated with the MHC molecules on APCs or target cells (e.g., virus-infected cell). Upon recognition of presented antigen, the T lymphocyte becomes activated and secretes cytokines (interleukins).

T Helper Lymphocytes

T helper lymphocytes (Th) are the primary regulators of delayed-type hypersensitivity responses. They express the CD4 molecule and regulate antigen-directed effector functions involved in cell-mediated immunity to pathogens. They also assist in the stimulation of B lymphocytes to proliferate and differentiate to become antibody-producing cells. T helper lymphocytes recognize foreign antigen complexed with MHC class II molecules on dendritic cells, on B cells, and on macrophages or other antigen-presenting cells that can express MHC class II.

T-Cytotoxic Lymphocytes

T-cytotoxic lymphocytes (CTLs) are cytotoxic against tumor cells and host cells infected with intracellular pathogens.

These cells usually express CD8 and destroy infected cells in an antigen-specific manner that is dependent upon the expression of MHC class I molecules that are expressed on almost all nucleated cells in the body. *T suppressor cells* express CD8 molecules and are thought to be related to CTLs. The suppressor cells function to suppress and limit T and B lymphocyte specific responses.

Natural Killer Cells

NK cells are large granular lymphocytes that kill tumor cells and virus-infected targets. NK cells share many surface molecules with T lymphocytes but do not express antigen-specific receptors such as the TCR/CD3 complex. Instead, NK cells express a variety of killer immunoglobulin-like receptors (KIRs), which can bind MHC class I molecules on target cells and send either a positive or negative signal for NK cell activation. NK cells adhere to infected target cells and induce their cell death via delivery of apoptic signals mediated by perforins, granzymes, and tumor necrosis factor alpha (TNF-α), or by effector interactions via their surface Fas ligand molecule with Fas on the target cell. NK cells can also kill through ADCC mechanisms via cell surface receptors for constant domains present on immunoglobulins.

●●● PRIMARY AND SECONDARY LYMPHOID ORGANS

The lymphatic organs are tissues in which leukocytes of myeloid and lymphoid origin mature, differentiate, and proliferate (Fig. 2-2). Lymphoid organs are composed of epithelial and stromal cells arranged either into discretely capsulated organs or accumulations of diffuse lymphoid tissue. The *primary (central) lymphoid organs* are the major sites of lymphopoiesis, e.g., where B and T lymphocytes differentiate from stem cells into mature antigen-recognizing cells. The *secondary lymphoid organs* are those tissues in which antigen-driven proliferation and differentiation occur.

Historically, the primary lymphoid organ was discovered in birds, in which B lymphocytes undergo maturation in the bursa of Fabricius, an organ situated near the cloaca. Humans do not have a cloaca, nor do they possess a bursa of Fabricius. In embryonic life, B lymphocytes mature and differentiate from hematopoietic stem cells in the fetal liver. After birth, B cells differentiate in the bone marrow. Maturation of T lymphocytes occurs in a different manner. Progenitor cells

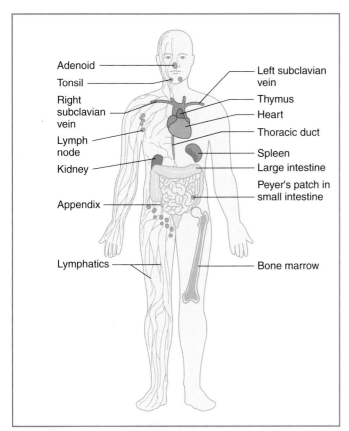

Figure 2-2. Distribution of lymphoid tissues.

Adenoid

Tonsil

Right subclavian vein

Lymph node

Kidney

Appendix

Lymphatics

Left subclavian vein

Thymus

Heart

Thoracic duct

Spleen

Large intestine

Peyer's patch in small intestine

Bone marrow

ANATOMY & EMBRYOLOGY

Ontogenic Development of Lymphoid Cells

Lymphocyte stem cells are produced first by the omentum and later by the yolk sac or fetal liver. In older fetuses and adults, the bone marrow is the major source of lymphocytes derived from pluripotent hematopoietic stem cells.

from the bone marrow migrate to the thymus, where they differentiate into T lymphocytes. The T lymphocytes continue to differentiate after leaving the thymus, and are driven to do so by encounter with APCs presenting trapped circulating antigen in the secondary lymphoid organs.

Primary Lymphoid Organs

Fetal Liver and Adult Bone Marrow

Islands or foci of hemopoietic progenitor cells in the fetal liver and in the adult bone marrow give rise directly to polymorphonuclear cells, monocytes, dendritic cells, B lymphocytes, and precursor T lymphocytes. Although the bone marrow is technically a primary lymphoid organ, recircula-

tion due to vascularization enables entry of circulating leukocytes from peripheral tissue, thereby also allowing bone marrow to serve a secondary lymphoid organ function.

Thymus Gland

The principal function of the thymus gland is to educate T lymphocytes to differentiate between self and non-self antigens. The thymus reaches maturity prior to puberty, with slow loss of function thereafter. This lymphoepithelial organ is primarily composed of stroma (thymic epithelium) and cells of the T lymphocyte lineage (Fig. 2-3). The thymus is divided into lobules containing cortex and medulla regions. Precursor T lymphocytes (*thymocytes*) differentiate to express specific receptors for antigen. The cortex contains immature thymocytes with few macrophages. The maturing lymphocytes pass through the medulla, interacting with epithelial cells, dendritic cells, and macrophages. Only 5% to 10% of thymocytes leave the thymus for final maturation in secondary organs. Hassal's corpuscles are a characteristic morphologic feature located within the medullary region of the thymus.

Secondary Lymphoid Organs

The secondary lymphoid organs provide localized environments where lymphocytes may respond to pathogens and foreign antigens. The spleen and lymph nodes are the major secondary lymphoid organs. Additional secondary lymphoid organs include the mucosa-associated lymphoid tissue (MALT), composed of cellular aggregates in the lamina propria of the digestive tract lining and respiratory tract.

Spleen

The spleen is a filter for blood that is histologically composed of two tissue types, red pulp and white pulp. The red pulp is made up of vascular sinusoids containing large numbers of macrophages, and is actively involved in the removal of dying and dead erythrocytes and of infectious agents (Fig. 2-4). The white pulp contains the lymphoid tissue, arranged around a central arteriole as a periarteriolar lymphoid sheath (PALS). The PALS is composed of T- and B-cell areas and follicles containing germinal centers. Dendritic reticular cells and phagocytic macrophages found in germinal centers present antigen to lymphocytes. The germinal centers are where B cells are stimulated to become plasma cells that produce and secrete antibodies.

Lymph Node

Lymph nodes (Fig. 2-5) form part of the lymphatic network that filters antigen and debris from lymph during its passage from the periphery to the thoracic duct. The *lymphatic vessels* (or lymphatics) are a network of thin tubes that branch into tissues throughout the body. Lymphatic vessels carry a colorless, watery fluid called *lymph*, which originates from interstitial fluid. Plasma and leukocytes from vascular tissue and capillary beds continuously circulate via afferent lymphatics, eventually arriving at draining lymph nodes. Histolo-

Figure 2-3. The thymus. Visible here are lobules with a darker staining cortex and a lighter staining medulla. The medulla is characterized by the presence of Hassall's corpuscles.

Labels in figure:
- Major Organs of the Immune System (Thymus)
- Capsule
- Cortical epithelial cell
- Trabecula
- Cortex
- Thymocyte
- Subcapsular epithelium
- Medullary epithelial cell
- Corticomedullary junction
- Dendritic cell
- Medulla
- Macrophage
- Hassall's corpuscle

gically, the lymph node is composed of an outer sinuous connective capsule. Subcapsular afferent vessels deliver antigen-containing fluid and draining pathogens into discrete lobules, where they are phagocytosed by antigen-presenting macrophages and dendritic cells. Naïve T lymphocytes enter the lymph node through specialized high endothelial venules and travel to the paracortex, where they encounter the APCs. A B lymphocyte–rich cortex contains both primary and secondary follicles and active germinal centers representing regions of lymphocyte division, differentiation, and expansion. Activated and memory lymphocytes eventually migrate through the central medullary sinus, leaving through efferent lymphatic vessels.

Mucosa-Associated Lymphoid Tissue (MALT)

Multiple nodules of partially encapsulated lymphoid tissue and loosely associated lymphoid aggregates are found in epithelia and lamina propria of mucosal surfaces (Fig. 2-6). Collectively, these aggregates located along the gastrointestinal and respiratory tracts are referred to as mucosa-associated lymphoid tissue (MALT), which can be further classified as gut-associated lymphoid tissue (GALT) or

Major Organs of the Immune System (Spleen)

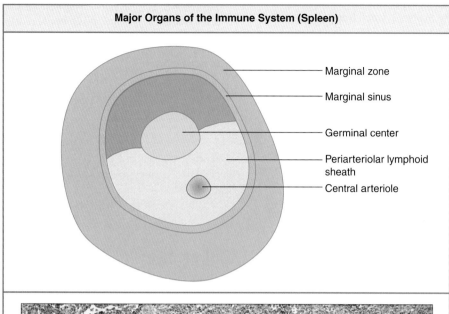

- Marginal zone
- Marginal sinus
- Germinal center
- Periarteriolar lymphoid sheath
- Central arteriole

Figure 2-4. The spleen. The white pulp of the spleen contains a central artery and associated follicle (germinal center, marginal zone, and periarteriolar lymphoid sheath).

bronchus-associated lymphoid tissue (BALT). The tonsils, appendix, and Peyer's patches are representative of lymphoid tissue found in and around mucosal epithelia. In particular, specialized microfold (M) cells of the follicle-associated epithelium of the MALT in gut and the respiratory system play a critical role in the genesis of immune responses by delivering foreign (non-host) material to underlying lymphoid tissue. Specialized resident intraepithelial lymphocytes (IELs) with potent cytolytic and immunoregulatory capacities monitor mucosal tissue to help defend against pathogenic infection.

KEY POINTS ABOUT CELLS AND ORGANS OF THE IMMUNE SYSTEM

- Physical barriers and biochemical mechanisms comprise the first line of defense against foreign pathogens. Once inside the body, innate and cellular components are required to fight infection.

- Innate cells and components are present from birth and represent a nonspecific first line of defense to foreign substances.

- Stem cell progenitors within the bone marrow are the precursors to myeloid and lymphoid progenitors, giving rise to

Major Organs of the Immune System (Lymph Node)

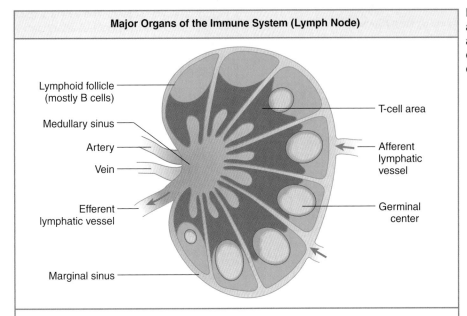

Lymphoid follicle (mostly B cells)

Medullary sinus

Artery

Vein

Efferent lymphatic vessel

Marginal sinus

T-cell area

Afferent lymphatic vessel

Germinal center

Figure 2-5. Lymph node. The normal architecture of a lymph node containing afferent and efferent lymphatic vessels, T cell–rich paracortex, and germinal centers of activation.

cells involved in either innate or adaptive immune responses. Myeloid cells include neutrophils, eosinophils, basophils, mast cells, monocytes, macrophages and dendritic cells. Lymphoid progenitors give rise to B and T lymphocytes and natural killer cells.

- Acquired (adaptive) immune responses discriminate between self and non-self and demonstrate specificity, memory, and adaptiveness. Humoral immunity refers to B lymphocytes, which produce antibodies that neutralize pathogens and toxins. Cellular immunity encompasses T lymphocytes to eradicate intracellular organisms.

- Primary lymphoid organs, such as the bone marrow and thymus, are the major sites of lymphopoiesis and where lymphocytes differentiate. Secondary lymphoid organs, such as the spleen and lymph nodes, are locations within the body where antigen-driven proliferation and maturation of lymphocytes occur. MALT (mucosa-associated lymphoid tissue) is loosely associated lymphoid aggregates where APCs located in the mucosal epithelia present antigens to lymphocytes.

Figure 2-6. Mucosa-associated lymphoid tissue (MALT). The tonsils (**A**), Peyer's patches (**B**), and appendix (**C**) all contain submucosal cellular aggregates representing lymphoid follicles, many with germinal centers.

Humoral Immunity: Antibody Recognition of Antigen

3

Humoral immunity refers to the arm of the acquired immune system that is mediated by antibody (immunoglobulin) recognition of antigens associated with foreign substances or pathogens. Antigen recognition is coupled with the ability to initiate biological responses that protect against microorganisms and neutralize viruses. The specific recognition of foreign antigen by B lymphocytes occurs through membrane-bound receptors and triggers proliferation and differentiation into antibody-producing plasma cells.

●●● ANTIBODY STRUCTURE AND FUNCTION

Antibody Is a Tetramer of Two Pairs of Identical Heavy and Light Chains

The antibody is a tetrameric polypeptide structure with distinct biological activity attributed to each end of the molecule (Fig. 3-1). Antibodies are composed of two identical heavy chain and two identical light chain polypeptides. Both heavy and light chain molecules have variable and constant domains and interact via intra- and inter-disulfide linkages. The variable region, termed $F(ab')_2$ (fragment, antibody binding) confers antigen recognition. The constant region, termed Fc (fragment, crystalline), interacts with cell surface receptors. The heavy chain contains a hinge domain that confers flexibility to allow optimal binding to antigen.

Antibodies Are Classified According to Their Heavy Chains

The constant regions of the heavy chain confer antibody function, representing five different classes, or *isotypes* (Fig. 3-2). Each class of heavy chain has a characteristic amino acid sequence that distinguishes it from the other four classes, but all five classes have a significant percentage of amino acid sequence similarities. The isotypes, IgM, IgD, IgG, IgE, and IgA, have characteristic properties (Table 3-1). The different heavy chains corresponding to their class are given Greek letter designations: γ, α, μ, ε, and δ. In many species, there are two or more subclasses of some heavy chains that differ from one another by only a few amino acids; humans have nine possible heavy chains each with unique biological functions. There are four subclasses of the IgG isotype, called IgG_1, IgG_2, IgG_3, and IgG_4, as listed in Table 3-2. IgA has two subclasses called IgA_1 and IgA_2.

Light chains come in two varieties, called kappa (κ) and lambda (λ). The difference between the two types of light chains is in the amino acid sequence of the constant region domain. The overall ratio of the two light chain types in human immunoglobulin is approximately 60% κ and 40% λ.

Both heavy and light chains have functional domains—amino acid sequences giving regularity to structure by way of disulfide-bridged loops. There are two domains on both κ and λ light chains and either four or five domains on heavy chains. The amino acid sequences in the first domain on both light and heavy chains are highly variant from molecule to molecule and are referred to as the variable light domain (V_L) or variable heavy domain (V_H). The light chain domain, which is constant in its amino acid sequence for the κ or λ type of

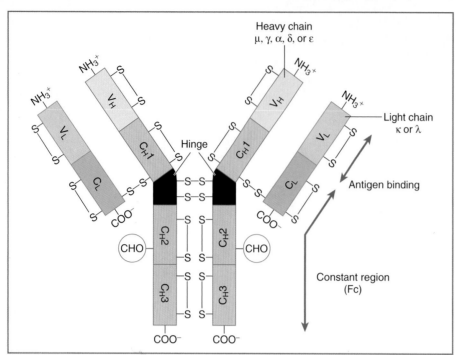

Figure 3-1. Antibody structure and functional domains. The basic structure of the antibody contains heavy chains and light chains, showing intra- and inter-disulfide bonds and the characteristic hinge region. The interactions between variable domains constitute the antigen-binding domain, while the constant regions confer specific biological properties to the molecule. CHO, carbohydrate.

Figure 3-2. Classes of antibody isotypes. Pictured are the five classes of antibody isotypes representing monomeric IgG, IgD, and IgE, pentameric IgM, and dimeric IgA with secretory component.

TABLE 3-1. Classes of Antibody Isotypes and Functional Properties*

Isotype	Immunoglobulin Class				
	IgM	IgD	IgG	IgE	IgA
Structure	Pentamer	Monomer	Monomer	Monomer	Monomer, dimer
Heavy chain designation	μ	δ	γ	ε	α
Molecular weight (kDa)	970	184	146–165	188	160 × 2
Serum concentration (mg/mL)	1.5	0.03	0.5–10.0	<0.0001	0.5–3.0
Serum half-life (days)	5–10	3	7–23	2.5	6
J chain	Yes	No	No	No	Yes
Complement activation	Strong	No	Yes, except IgG_4	No	No
Bacterial toxin neutralization	Yes	No	Yes	No	Yes
Antiviral activity	No	No	Yes	No	Yes
Binding to mast cells and basophils	No	No	No	Yes	No
Additional properties	Effective agglutinator of particulate antigens, bacterial opsonization	Found on surface of mature B cells, signaling via cytoplasmic tail	Antibody-dependent cell cytotoxicity	Mediation of allergic response, effective against parasitic worms	Monomer in secretory fluid, active as dimer on epithelial surfaces

*Refer also to Figure 3-2.

TABLE 3-2. Unique Biological Properties of Human IgG Subclasses

	IgG_1	IgG_2	IgG_3	IgG_4
Occurrence (% of total IgG)	70	20	7	3
Half-life (days)	23	23	7	23
Complement binding	+	+	Strong	No
Placental passage	++	±	++	++
Receptor binding to monocytes	Strong	+	Strong	±

BIOCHEMISTRY

Amino Acid Protein Structure

The combination of disulfide links between cysteine residues and the proline-rich hinge region gives the antibody molecule the unique structure and flexibility necessary to interact with antigens.

chain, is referred to as the C_L domain. The constant domains of heavy chains are numbered from the amino terminal to the carboxyl terminal as C_H1, C_H2, C_H3, and (for IgM and IgE) C_H4.

IgG, IgA, and IgD genes each have an exon coding for a short span of amino acids that occupy the space between the C_H1 and C_H2 domains. This segment is rich in cysteine and proline and permits significant flexibility between the two arms of the antibody; the area is called the *hinge region*. This stretch is highly susceptible to protease cleavage.

Vertebrates and invertebrates express a large number of closely related cell-surface proteins, many of which appear to have evolved from common gene sequences. Collectively, they are called the immunoglobulin gene superfamily. All members of the immunoglobulin gene superfamily contain structures called Ig (immunoglobulin) domains, which share the primary amino acid sequence and physical structure of β-pleated sheets with intrachain disulfide bonds. Members

of the Ig gene superfamily include surface receptors and adhesion molecules.

●●● ANTIBODY-ANTIGEN INTERACTIONS

Antigen Binding Occurs in the Antibody Variable Region Domain

The molecular conformation in the variable region of an antibody that confers antigenic specificity is referred to as the *idiotype*; the site of direct contact in the variable region is called the *paratope*. Each antibody molecule can bind between two and 10 antigenic determinants (as long as they are physically close together), depending on the number of available F(ab) regions present. IgG, IgD, and IgE have two F(ab) binding sites. IgA as a dimer has four binding sites; the pentameric IgM molecule has 10 binding sites. An aggregated antigen with multiple repeating epitopes (such as those found in bacterial capsules or carbohydrate ABO blood groups)

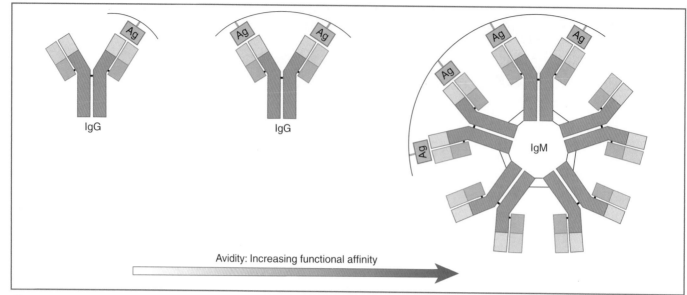

Figure 3-3. Multivalent interactions increase functional affinity of antibody-antigen-binding. Interactions of repeating antigens with more than one functional antigen-binding region allows greater stabilization of binding and increases functional affinity. Monomeric IgG can bind either one or two epitopes, whereas pentameric IgM can bind up to 10. Ag, antigen.

allows increase in total binding strength, thereby raising the overall *avidity* (or *functional affinity*) of the interaction (Fig. 3-3).

Physiochemical Forces Are Involved in Antigen-Antibody Interactions

Antibodies can bind a wide variety of molecules with high specificity, ranging from large macromolecules to small chemical moieties. The molecular region on the antigen recognized by immune components is called an *epitope*, or *antigenic determinant*. Antibody-binding to antigen does not involve covalent chemical bonds. The strength of binding to epitopes on the antigen, or the interaction affinity, is based on multiple forces present within the binding site (Fig. 3-4).

● ● ● ANTIGENS AND IMMUNOGENS

An antigen is any substance that can be recognized by the immune system. Major classes of antigens include proteins,

carbohydrates, lipids, and nucleic acids. In contrast, an *immunogen* is any substance that can evoke an immune response. Not all antigens are immunogenic. For example, *haptens* are low-molecular-weight compounds that are nonimmunogenic by themselves but are antigenic; haptens become immunogenic after conjugation to high-molecular-weight immunogenic carriers. The rule to remember is that *all immunogens are antigens, but not all antigens are immunogens*. This concept is important when considering rational design of vaccines.

Antibodies Recognize Both Sequential and Conformational Epitopes

Two general classes of epitopes can be distinguished on antigens. They are best described as they exist on protein antigens, but other classes of antigens (e.g., carbohydrates and nucleic acids) can exhibit both under some circumstances. *Sequential epitopes* are short stretches of amino acids (4–7 in length) that can be recognized by antibodies when the short peptide exists free in solution or when it is chemically coupled to another protein molecule. *Conformational epitopes* require the native three-dimensional configuration of the molecule to be intact, and antigenic determinants need not be contiguous; denaturation of the molecule destroys these kinds of epitopes.

Cross-Reactivity Occurs When Antigens Share Similar Structure

The forces mediating antigen-antibody recognition allow for a high degree of specificity. That is, antibodies specific for one epitope or hapten can easily distinguish that epitope or hapten from other similar structures. This specificity is not absolute; antibodies specific for one epitope can bind with

BIOCHEMISTRY

Noncovalent Bond Forces

The weak interactions represented by noncovalent bond forces are important in multiple biological systems, allowing for fluidity of information, as seen with ligands interacting with cellular receptors. One of these interactions is the van der Waals forces, which are relatively weak electric forces that attract neutral atoms and molecules to one another in gases, in liquefied and solidified gases, and in almost all organic liquids and solids. These forces arise from polarization induced in each particle by the presence of other particles.

Major antigen (AG) classes
Carbohydrates
Polysaccharides
Proteins
Glycoproteins
Nucleic acids
Lipids

Requirements for immunogenicity
Physiochemical complexity
Molecular weight > 6 kDa
Foreignness (non-self)
Degradability

Figure 3-4. Noncovalent forces contribute to avidity of antibody-antigen interactions. Binding of antigen to antibody is a noncovalent interaction. The major forces involved are depicted.

MICROBIOLOGY

Antibacterial Vaccines

Group B streptococcus causes invasive infections of newborns and adults, with commonly reported bacteremia, meningitis, and pneumonia. The associated polysaccharide capsule antigens are being targeted for use in vaccines, utilizing methods that conjugate carbohydrates to a protein carrier to create T-dependent antigens.

BIOCHEMISTRY

Gene Transcription and RNA Translation

The production of protein involves gene transcription of DNA into primary RNA transcripts by polymerases, under control of transcription factors. The primary transcript is further processed by splicing out noncoding introns, to produce full messenger RNA (mRNA), which is eventually translated into protein. In B lymphocytes, the zinc finger transcription factor early growth response 1 (*Egr-1*) is one of the many immediate-early genes induced upon B-cell antigen receptor engagement.

---

structurally similar nonidentical epitopes with a lower affinity. *Cross-reactivity* refers to the situation in which an antibody can react with two similar molecules because they share one or more identical epitope or the epitope in question is similar enough in sequence or shape to bind with weaker affinity. For example, antibodies elicited with toxoids react with native toxins, allowing clinical application for vaccination with nonpathogenic antigens like tetanus toxoid and diphtheria toxoid.

●●● GENETIC BASIS OF ANTIBODY STRUCTURE

The generation of antigen-binding capability of the antibody B-cell receptor occurs prior to antigen exposure through DNA rearrangement involving combinations of multiple genes to achieve high diversity needed for immune responses. Recombination occurs for both heavy and light chain genes by way of an enzyme complex known as *V(D)J recombinase*. The recombinase is the product of two genes (*RAG-1* and *RAG-2*; recombinase-activating genes); defects in either *RAG-1* or *RAG-2* can cause a spectrum of severe immunodeficiencies with devastating clinical complications.

The organization of heavy chain genes shows three different regions contributing to production of the variable region. These gene segments are referred to as V_H (variable), D_H (diversity), and J_H (joining) (Fig. 3-5). There are approx-

imately 50 V_H genes, 20 D_H genes, and up to 6 J_H genes present in germline DNA. The V(D)J recombinase mediates joining of different gene segments through mechanisms by which intervening segments are spliced out of the genome within that particular B cell. This process requires pairing of 7-base-pair and 9-base-pair gene sequences, after which the intervening DNA is "looped out" and deleted permanently from the chromosome. To complete the process, alternative splicing brings the rearranged VDJ sequence together with distinct gene segments coding for the C_H (constant) region.

Similar events occur for rearrangement of the light chain locus. In humans (and most other mammals) there are two light chain loci—κ and λ—located on different chromosomes. The germline arrangement for light chains is similar to that of the heavy chain locus, except there are no D gene segments. In addition, for the κ locus there is only one constant region, whereas the λ locus has multiple constant regions, each with its own J gene segment.

●●● GENERATION OF ANTIBODY DIVERSITY

The portions of the variable region that participate in antigen-binding are called *complementarity-determining regions* (CDRs). Amino acids in these hypervariable regions contact

Figure 3-5. Genetic organization and recombination events. Antibody diversity is generated by DNA recombination events that randomly fuse variable, diversity, and joining regions. The recombination is accomplished in a defined order by enzymes RAG-1 and RAG-2. The first events culminate in transcribing mRNA coding for IgM and IgD; differential translation determines whether mature polypeptide will be IgM or IgD. L, leader sequence; V, variable; D, diversity; J, joining; C, constant region.

residues for antigen; the CDRs form the region of structural complementarity for antigenic epitopes, and differences in antigen-binding are due to differences in these sequences. Two of the CDRs (CDR1 and CDR2) are "hard-wired" into the V gene segment and thus depend upon the V segment selected during rearrangement. CDR3 consists of the junction of the V, D, and J gene segments and hence has a high degree of variability. The CDRs of both the heavy and light chain participate in the formation of the antigen-binding pocket (paratope).

Four major mechanisms for generating antibody diversity in humans occur during B-cell development, before antigen exposure. These mechanisms give rise to a repertoire of antibodies that in theory have the capability of recognizing approximately 10^{14} different epitopes.

Multiple Variable Gene Segments

There are greater than 50 V gene segments in the heavy chain locus and approximately 40 V gene segments each in the κ light chain loci and nearly as many V gene segments in the λ loci.

Combinatorial Diversity

The V, D, and J regions in heavy chains (and the V and J regions in light chains) are selected randomly during V(D)J rearrangement ("joining"). Thus, 50 V_H genes × 26 D_H genes × 6 J_H genes yields more than 6000 possible heavy chain VDJ

loci combinations. A lesser degree of variation occurs in the light chain recombination, because there are no D regions; there are about 200 and about 160 different VJ combinations in κ and λ, respectively.

Heavy and Light Chain Combinations

Because the heavy and light chain loci recombine independently, each B cell will contain a different combination of randomly assorted heavy and light chains.

Junctional and Insertional Diversity

The recombination between V and D-J segments and between D and J segments is not precise, often staggering the junctional location between recombined segments by a few base pairs. This "sloppiness" causes differences in the amino acid sequence and leads to junctional diversity. Insertional diversity results from the activity of terminal deoxynucleotide transferase (TdT), an enzyme that is expressed during heavy chain rearrangement. TdT adds nucleotides randomly at the V-D and D-J junctions.

●●● ISOTYPE SWITCHING AND AFFINITY MATURATION

Secretion of antibodies occurs only after antigenic stimulation of membrane-anchored immunoglobulin on the B-cell surface. Differentiation into plasma cells usually occurs in

Figure 3-6. Isotype class switching. During plasma cell differentiation, the antibody isotype may be changed where the same variable region is recombined with a different constant region gene sequence. Intervening DNA is excised, allowing generation of mRNA for different isotypes. Subsequent switching may occur to any downstream remaining coding sequence; however, once done, the change is irreversible.

germinal centers of lymph nodes, the spleen, or MALT-associated tissue. The process requires both antigenic recognition and help given in the form of T-cell cytokines. During differentiation, two processes can occur to change the biological properties of the secreted antibody. The first is class switching, or *isotype switching*, in which deletion of intervening DNA sequences occurs, allowing antibodies to switch from IgM and IgD to another isotype (Fig. 3-6).

Isotype switching results when antigen-stimulated B cells receive a cytokine signal from T helper cells. The V region does not change during isotype switching; therefore, the same antigenic specificity is retained. Switching involves the deletion of intervening DNA between specific recombination sites called switch regions. Because the intervening DNA is lost, the B cell cannot "switch back" to an isotype that has already been deleted. The V region and C regions are transcribed together, and RNA splicing and translation results in expression of the *new* isotype.

The second process is termed *affinity maturation*, in which germline DNA is subject to mutational change allowing coding for antibodies with increased affinity for binding to antigen. This process is a result of somatic hypermutation in which V regions of the antibody heavy and light chain genes undergo a more than 10,000 times higher rate of mutation than "regular" DNA. Somatic hypermutation occurs only after antigen stimulation. Some of these mutations increase the affinity of antibody for antigen, and those B cells express-

ing antibody with higher affinity will be selectively stimulated, increasing the proportion of high-affinity antibody in secondary responses.

KEY POINTS ABOUT HUMORAL IMMUNITY

- The basic immunoglobulin (antibody) unit consists of two light and two heavy chains, all covalently bound via disulfide bridges. Domains of the molecule are responsible for unique biological functions.

- There are five classes or isotypes of heavy chains—γ, α, μ, δ, and ε—corresponding to the heavy chains of IgG, IgA, IgM, IgD, and IgE, respectively. There are two types of light chains in humans—κ and λ—distinguished by different amino acid sequences in the constant domain.

- Antibodies recognize antigenic determinants (epitopes); the major classes of antigens include proteins or glycoproteins, nucleic acids, carbohydrates, and lipids.

- Antibody-binding to antigen occurs in hypervariable regions and does not utilize covalent interactions. Multiple weak forces stabilize the binding, including electrostatic interactions, hydrogen bonding, hydrophobic interactions, and van der Waals forces.

- Generation of antigen-binding diversity results from V(D)J recombination during B-cell development and somatic mutation after antigenic stimulation. Biofunctional diversity of antibodies results from isotype switching, with unique biofunctions associated with each antibody isotype. Each individual B cell and all of its progeny express only one heavy chain and one light chain V region sequence, and thus all have the same antigenic specificity.

- There are multiple sources of antibody diversity: (1) presence of multiple V gene segments; (2) combinatorial diversity, resulting from random recombination of V, D, and J segment combinations; (3) junctional and insertional diversity, resulting in changes in the V-D and D-J junctions; (4) coexpression of different heavy and light chain pairs; and (5) somatic hypermutation.

T-Cell Immunity

4

A

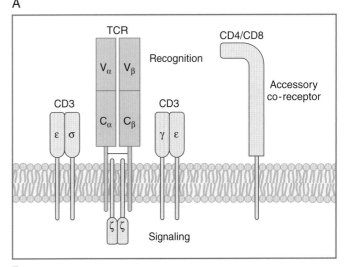

B

Figure 4-1. Structure of the TCR complex. **A**, The structure of the T-cell receptor (TCR) complex showing the predominant form of the antigen-binding chains, α (40–50 kDa) and β (35–47 kDa). A T cell expresses a TCR of only one specificity. Both transmembrane peptides exhibit two external domains connected via a disulfide bridging bond. A hydrophobic helical domain crosses the cellular membrane, leaving a short cytoplasmic tail. **B**, The TCR is always expressed with the associated CD3 complex, required for signal transduction, composed of γ, δ, and ε chains plus two ζ chains. T_H cells express CD4, required for interaction with antigen presenting cells, whereas cytotoxic T cells express the CD8 coreceptor molecule. CHO, carbohydrate

Thymus-dependent T lymphocytes are involved in regulation of immune response and cell-mediated immunity. Overall, they regulate the major properties of the acquired immune response leading to specificity of antigenic recognition and discrimination between self and non-self. There are two major classes of T cells; helper T cells and cytotoxic T cells (CTLs). T helper (T_H) cells are further divided into classes that assist in the activation of antigen-presenting cells to kill intracellular bacteria or to help B cells produce antibody. CTLs primarily target virally infected cells and tumor cells.

●●● ANTIGEN-SPECIFIC RECEPTORS

Mature T cells express T-cell receptors (TCRs) specific for antigen (Fig. 4-1). The TCR is expressed on the cell surface in association with coreceptors and accessory molecules that allow T cells to recognize presented antigens associated with the major histocompatibility complex (MHC) molecules on target cells. The TCR is a transmembrane heterodimer composed of two disulfide-linked polypeptide chains. T cells of all antigenic specificities exist prior to contact with antigen. Each lymphocyte carries a TCR of only a single specificity, which when stimulated by antigen, gives rise to progeny with identical antigenic specificity.

The vast majority of peripheral T cells express alpha (α) and beta (β) chains on their surface. Cells that express gamma (γ) and delta (δ) chains make up only 5% of the normal circulating T-cell population in healthy adults. Each chain (α,β,γ, or δ) represents a distinct protein with approximate molecular weight of 45 kDa. An individual T cell can express

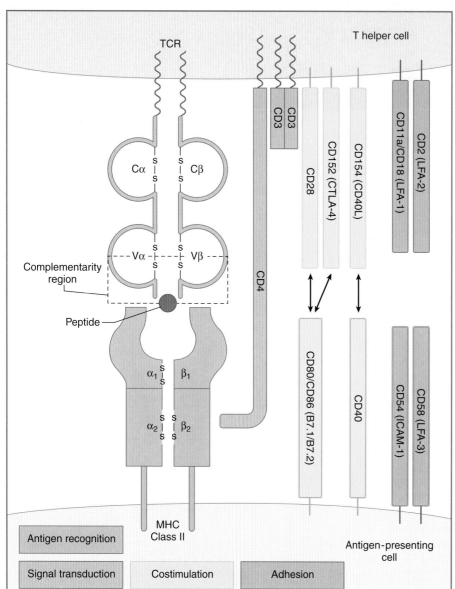

Figure 4-2. Interaction of TCR, MHC, and peptide. The complementarity determining regions (CDRs) of the TCR variable regions and peptide bound in the binding groove of an MHC class II molecule are depicted. The TCR recognizes portions of both the MHC molecule and the bound antigen. For T$_H$ cells, recognition of the presented antigen is enhanced by CD4, which attaches to nonpolymorphic regions on the MHC molecule. Further stabilization is accomplished by integrin interactions between molecules on the T cell with ligands on the surface of the APC. Costimulatory molecules present on both the T cell and the APC are critical for T-cell function and activation.

either an αβ or a γδ heterodimer as its receptor, but never both.

The TCR recognizes antigen in the form of short linear peptides that are bound in an antigen-binding pocket, or "groove," in the MHC molecules. The interactions between the TCR heterodimers create three hypervariable regions called complementarity determining regions (CDRs 1, 2, and 3), which confer specificity for antigen recognition (Fig. 4-2). The TCR heterodimer is in tight noncovalent association with the CD3 complex, made up of independently encoded subunits (one δ, γ, ε, and two ζ). The CD3 complex is required for efficient transport of the TCR to the cell surface. CD3 subunits possess long intracellular tails and are responsible for transducing signals upon TCR engagement of antigen in the context of MHC. Other coreceptors enhance the ability of T cells to respond to antigen; CD4 molecules assist helper cell interactions, while CD8 molecules contribute to CTL activity,

both by binding to invariant regions of MHC class II and I molecules (see Chapter 5), respectively, on adjacent cells. Numerous molecules on the T-cell surface, including integrin cell adhesion molecules and the Ig family member CD28, promote T-cell adhesion to target cells or APCs (facilitating antigen recognition) and provide necessary costimulatory signals that further drive T-cell responses.

KEY POINTS ABOUT T LYMPHOCYTES

- T lymphocytes are involved in regulation of immune response and in cell-mediated immunity.

- Mature T cells express antigen-specific TCR in a complex with CD3 molecules. The TCR is a disulfide-linked heterodimer composed of either αβ or γδ chains. T cells express either αβ or γδ chain heterodimers, but never both.

●●● GENES CODING FOR T-CELL RECEPTORS

Genes that code for the T-cell receptor and the mechanisms used to generate TCR diversity are similar to those of immunoglobulins. In fact, the T-cell receptor genes are closely related members of the immunoglobulin gene superfamily. Each chain consists of a constant (C) and a variable (V) region. The repertoire is generated by combinatorial joining of variable (V), joining (J), and diversity (D) genes and by N region diversification (nucleotides inserted by the enzyme deoxynucleotidyl transferase) (Fig. 4-3). Unlike immunoglobulin genes, genes encoding TCR do not undergo somatic mutation. Thus, there is no change in the affinity of the TCR during activation, differentiation, and expansion.

The TCR V, D, and J genes are mixed together in a more complicated manner than found for immunoglobulin genes. For example, the α and γ chains use only V and J gene segments, whereas the β and δ chains use V, D, and J gene segments. There are many more Vα and Vβ genes (50–100) than Vγ and Vδ genes (5–10) present in germline. The α and δ chain genes are mixed together in one locus. The genes encoding the δ chain are located entirely between the cluster of Vα and Jα gene segments.

Recombination of V, D, and J gene segments is coordinated by recombinase-activating genes *RAG-1* and *RAG-2*. The enzymes recognize specific DNA signal sequences consisting of a heptamer, followed by a spacer of 12 or 23 bases, and then a nonamer. If either *RAG* gene is impaired, mutated, or missing, homologous recombination events are abolished. This gives rise to severe combined immunodeficiency (SCID). An example of such a disorder is Omenn's syndrome, an

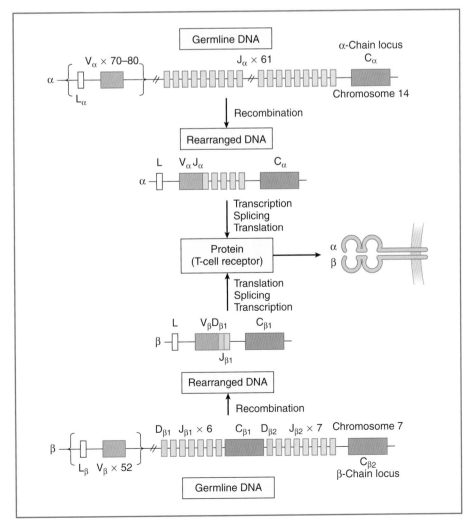

Figure 4-3. Gene rearrangement of T-cell receptor genes. TCR diversity is generated by combinatorial joining of variable (V), joining (J), and diversity (D) genes and by N region diversification (nucleotides inserted by the enzyme deoxynucleotidyl transferase). The top and bottom rows show germline arrangement of the V, D, J, and constant (C) gene segments at the T-cell receptor α and β loci. During T-cell development, a V region sequence for each chain is assembled by DNA recombination. For the α chain (top), a Vα gene segment rearranges to a Jα gene segment to create a functional gene encoding the V domain. For the β chain (bottom), rearrangement of a Dβ, a Jβ, and a Vβ gene segment creates the functional V domain exon.

autosomal recessive form of SCID characterized by high susceptibility to fungal, bacterial, and viral infections.

The order of gene rearrangement is sequential. An immature T lymphocyte entering the thymus has its TCR genes in the germline configuration, since rearrangement has not yet taken place. Both γ and β chain genes then begin to rearrange, more or less simultaneously. If the γ chain genes rearrange successfully, then δ chain genes also start to rearrange. If both γ and δ genes rearrange functionally, no further gene rearrangement takes place and the cell remains a γδ T cell. If γ and/or δ rearrangements are not functional, then β gene rearrangement continues followed by α gene rearrangement. In this manner, a αβ product appears, and the cell becomes an αβ T cell.

The overall level of diversity is greater for T-cell receptors than for immunoglobulins; up to 10^{18} possible antigen-specific T-cell receptors are generated compared with 10^{14} possible antibody specificities (Fig. 4-4). The increased T-cell diversity is due to additional junctional regions and greater N nucleotide addition during recombination, coding for regions corresponding to the CDR3 loops that form the center of antigen-binding sites. Although there is great variability in the binding-site regions, the remaining framework portion of the heterodimer is subject to relatively little variation.

KEY POINTS ABOUT T-CELL RECEPTOR GENES

- T-cell receptor genes are closely related members of the immunoglobulin gene superfamily and derive part of their structural diversity from recombination of different V, D, and J gene segments.

- The process of recombination is coordinated by recombinase-activating genes *RAG-1* and *RAG-2*.

- Unlike the B-cell antibody genes, T-cell receptor genes do not undergo somatic mutations.

PATHOLOGY

Severe Combined Immunodeficiency (SCID)

Lymph node biopsies in SCID patients with Omenn's syndrome demonstrate an absence of germinal centers and replacement of the paracortex by a diffuse infiltrate of large cells with abundant pale cytoplasm.

●●● DEVELOPMENT OF T LYMPHOCYTES

Progenitor cells from the bone marrow migrate to the thymus, where they differentiate into T lymphocytes (Fig. 4-5). In

Common Properties of TCR and Antibody
Integral membrane proteins
Thousands of identical copies at cell surface
Made before cell encounters antigen
Gene assembled by DNA recombination
Allelic exclusion for single antigenic specifity
N region addition during gene rearrangement
Antigen binding by noncovalent forces
Binding signals replication and activation

Properties Unique to TCR
Structure and encoding genes
Binding presented epitopes
Never secreted from the T cell
No somatic mutation
No isotype switching
High junctional diversity

	Immunoglobulins	T cell α:β Receptors
Number of V gene pairs	3.4×10^6	5.8×10^6
Junctional diversity	$\sim 3 \times 10^7$	$\sim 2 \times 10^{11}$
Total diversity	$\sim 10^{14}$	$\sim 10^{18}$

Figure 4-4. Comparison of diversity between B- and T-cell receptors.

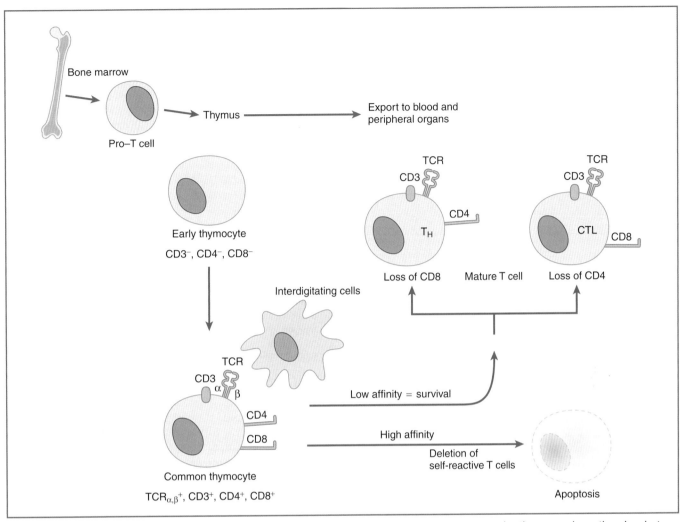

Figure 4-5. Main stages in thymic selection. Pro-T cells migrating from the bone marrow enter the thymus, where they begin to express rearranged TCR, CD3, CD4, and CD8 proteins. Positive selection occurs to eliminate self-reactive T cells, through mechanisms of apoptosis. Maturing thymocytes lose either CD4 or CD8 surface molecules, and they are exported to peripheral tissue as CD4$^+$ T$_H$ cells or as CD8$^+$ CTLs. T$_H$, T helper.

the thymus, immature T cells undergo rearrangement of their TCR genes to generate a diverse set of clonotypic TCRs. Immature thymocytes are selected for further maturation only if their TCRs do not interact with self-peptides presented in the context of self-MHC molecules on antigen-presenting cells. Positively selected thymocytes undergo commitment to either the T cytotoxic or T helper (T$_H$) lineages. Deletion of self-reactive T cells occurs through apoptosis. Lineage commitment is marked phenotypically by the loss of expression of one of the coreceptor molecules, CD8 or CD4. Immature thymocytes express both coreceptors (double positive), whereas T killer or T$_H$ cells express only CD8 or CD4, respectively (single positive CD8$^+$ or CD4$^+$). T lymphocytes continue to differentiate after leaving the thymus, driven by encounter with specific antigen in the secondary lymphoid organs (spleen, lymph nodes, and mucosa-associated lymphoid tissue).

Virtually all the cells that express the TCR-αβ are CD4$^+$ (T$_H$) or CD8$^+$ (T cytotoxic or T suppressor). Almost all cells

PHYSIOLOGY

Apoptosis

Apoptosis, or programmed cell death, is the regulated elimination of cells that occurs naturally during the course of development, as well as in many pathologic circumstances that require cell death for the benefit of the organism. For example, during vertebrate embryonic development, the notochord and the floor plate secrete a gradient of the signaling molecule Sonic hedgehog (Shh), which directs cells to form patterns in the embryonic neural tube.

expressing TCR-γδ are CD4$^-$ CD8$^-$ (double negative). Whereas the TCR-αβ-expressing lymphocytes are known to function as effector cells, the function of the TCR-γδ cells is not well understood.

Figure 4-6. Effector functions of T_H cells. T_H1 cells activate macrophages through production of cytokines, leading to assisted destruction of intracellular microorganisms. T_H2 cells drive B-cell differentiation to stimulate B cells to proliferate, to secrete immunoglobulins, and to undergo isotype switching events. IFN, interferon; IL, interleukin; TNF-α, tumor necrosis factor alpha.

TABLE 4-1. Characteristics of T Helper Cell Subsets

Cytokine Profile	T_H1	T_H2	T_H3
IL-2, TNF-β, IFN-γ	++++	−	±
IL-4, IL-5, IL-6, IL-10	−	++++	±
TGF-β	±	±	++++
IL-10	±	++	±
Growth factor	IL-2	IL-2/IL-4	IL-4/TGF-β
Effector function	Cellular immunity	B-cell maturation	Oral tolerance

IFN, interferon; IL, interleukin; TGF, transforming growth factor; TNF, tumor necrosis factor.

●●● UNIQUE EFFECTOR FUNCTIONS OF T-CELL PHENOTYPES

T Helper Cells

T_H cells are the primary regulators of T cell– and B cell–mediated responses (Fig. 4-6). They (1) aid antigen-stimulated subsets of B lymphocytes to proliferate and differentiate toward antibody-producing cells; (2) express the CD4 co-receptor molecule; (3) recognize foreign antigen complexed with MHC class II molecules on B cells, macrophages, or other antigen-presenting cells; and (4) aid effector T lymphocytes in cell-mediated immunity. There are three functional subsets of T_H cells, each demonstrating unique effector function (Table 4-1). T helper 1 (T_H1) cells aid in the regulation of cellular immunity. T helper 2 (T_H2) cells aid B cells to produce certain classes of antibodies (e.g., IgA and IgE). The third class of T helper cells (T_H3) is thought to be involved in oral tolerance and serves as regulators for mucosal immunity.

KEY POINTS ABOUT T HELPER LYMPHOCYTES

- T_H lymphocytes recognize specific Ag in the context of MHC class II on APCs. Although this is required for T-cell activation, it is not sufficient. Other accessory molecules on T cells, such as integrins and CD28, which bind counter-ligands on the adjacent

cell, promote firm adhesion between T cell and APC and send necessary secondary signals that fully activate T cells.

- Activation of the T_H cell leads to specific cytokine release; different classes of T_H cells secrete specific subsets of cytokines.

T Cytotoxic Cells

T cytotoxic cells (CTLs) are cytotoxic against tumor cells and host cells infected with intracellular pathogens (Fig. 4-7). These cells (1) express the CD8 coreceptor and (2) destroy infected cells in an antigen-specific manner that is dependent upon the expression of MHC class I molecules on antigen-presenting cells. CTLs are able to kill target cells directly by inducing apoptosis. Nucleases and other enzymes activated in the apoptotic process may help destroy the viral genome, thus preventing the assembly of virions and potential infection of other cells. CTLs induce apoptosis only in the target cell; neighboring tissue cells are not affected. Two mechanisms for induction of apoptosis have been identified. One method utilizes preformed perforins directionally released from the CTL to the target cell surface that generate transmembrane pores, through which a second group of proteins, granzymes, can gain entry to the cytosol and induce an apoptotic series of events. The other method occurs by apoptotic signaling via membrane-bound Fas molecules on the target cell surface and Fas ligand on the CTL surface. The processes of antigen recognition, CTL activation, and delivery of apoptotic signals to the target cell can be accomplished within 10 minutes. The apoptotic process in the targeted cell may take 4 hours or more and continues long after the CTL has moved on to interact with other potential targets.

KEY POINTS ABOUT T CYTOTOXIC CELLS

- CTLs recognize Ag in the context of MHC class I and, like T_H cells, are fully activated by accessory costimulatory molecules.
- CTLs kill target cells directly by inducing apoptosis. They release preformed perforins at the target cell surface to generate transmembrane pores in the target cell, through which a second

Figure 4-7. Effector function of cytotoxic T cells. CTLs recognize virally infected target cells which express foreign antigens complexed with MHC class I molecules. Cytotoxic effector molecules produced by the CTL initiate destruction of the target cell and delivery of apoptotic signals. $\beta_2 M$, β_2 microglobulin.

set of proteins and granzymes gain entry into the cytosol to initiate an apoptotic series of events.

- CTLs can also deliver apoptotic signals via surface-bound molecules.

T Regulatory/Suppressor Cells

It is thought that a group of lymphocytes exist with function to suppress the cellular (T cell) and humoral (B cell) responses. However, it is not entirely clear whether this group represents a separate subpopulation of CD4+ or CD8+ lymphocytes or merely reflects consequent activities of T cells that produce cytokines which down-regulate developmental pathways of T_H responsiveness. Recent work indicates that this population can express both the CD4 marker and the IL-2 receptor α chain (CD25) and requires specific engagement of the TCR for function.

●●● γδ T CELLS

γδ T cells are predominantly found in the lamina propria of the gut and are thought to assist in protection against microorganisms entering through epithelium at mucosal surfaces. Their range of response to antigens is limited. γδ-expressing cells have been found to be active toward mycobacterial antigens and heat shock proteins. The cells have the ability to secrete cytokines like their αβ counterparts. Generally, γδ cells lack CD4 and CD8 (double negative cells), although some γδ cells do express CD8. Some γδ T cells can function in the absence of MHC molecules.

Role of Major Histocompatibility Complex in the Immune Response

5

CONTENTS

●●● FUNCTION OF THE MAJOR HISTOCOMPATIBILITY COMPLEX (MHC)

The major histocompatibility complex (MHC) is a gene locus composed of multiple sequences that code for histocompatibility antigens. Histocompatibility antigens are cell surface glycoproteins that play critical roles in interactions among immune system cells. MHC genes are organized into two major classes. Class I gene products are found on all nucleated cells and participate in antigen presentation to CD8$^+$ cytotoxic lymphocytes (CTL). Class II molecules are found primarily on antigen-presenting cells (B cells, macrophages, and dendritic cells) and participate in antigen presentation by macrophages to CD4$^+$ lymphocytes (T$_H$ cells).

MHC genes are very polymorphic. In humans, the MHC locus is designated as the human leukocyte antigen (HLA) locus.

MHC molecules were so-named because they were first identified as the targets for rejection of grafts between individuals. When organs are transplanted between a donor and a recipient with MHC locus differences, graft rejection is prompt. The function of the MHC is the presentation of antigen fragments (epitopes) to T cells.

●●● ORGANIZATION AND HIGH POLYMORPHISM OF MHC GENES AND GENE PRODUCTS

The HLA locus in humans is found on the short arm of chromosome 6 (Fig. 5-1). The class I region consists of HLA-A, HLA-B, and HLA-C loci. The class II region consists of the D region, which is subdivided into HLA-DP, HLA-DQ, and HLA-DR subregions. A region between the class I and class II loci encodes for class II proteins with no structural similarity to either class I or class II molecules (complement proteins, tumor necrosis factor, and lymphotoxin).

The highly polymorphic class I and class II MHC products are central to the ability of T cells to recognize foreign antigen and the ability to discriminate "self" from "non-self." MHC class I and class II molecules that are not possessed by an individual are seen as foreign antigens upon transplantation and are dealt with accordingly by the recipient's immune system. All MHC molecules show a high level of allotypic polymorphism; i.e., certain regions of the molecules differ from one person to another. The chance of two unrelated people having the same allotypes at all genes that encode MHC molecules is very small.

The class I MHC molecules are each somewhat different from one another with respect to amino acid sequence, and all three (HLA-A, HLA-B, and HLA-C) are codominantly expressed in the membrane of every nucleated cell (as high as 5×10^5 molecules per cell on lymphocytes). "Codominantly expressed" means that each gene encoding these proteins from both parental chromosomes is expressed. MHC class I

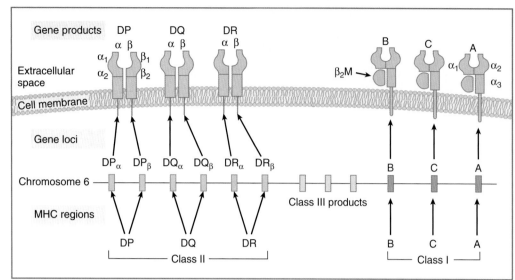

Figure 5-1. Genetic organization of the HLA locus and associated gene products. The polymorphic human MHC genes of the HLA locus coding for class I and class II molecules are located on chromosome 6. Class I genes are designated as A, B, and C, each coding for a three-domain polypeptide (α_1, α_2, α_3) that associates with invariant β_2-microglobulin. Class II genes are DP, DQ, and DR, each coding for individual α and β chains that interact to provide binding sites for antigen presentation.

molecules expressed on progeny (F1) cells match maternal or paternal class I molecules. The MHC class II molecules expressed on F1 cells include homologous and heterologous $\alpha\beta$ dimer mixtures, since both α and β subunit genes exhibit species-specific polymorphism. Homologous dimers match class II molecules expressed on either parental cell type, whereas heterologous dimers are unique to the F1 genotype and are functionally nonequivalent to parental class II molecules.

KEY POINTS ABOUT MHC GENES AND GENE PRODUCTS

- MHC molecules are important for antigen presentation to T cells.
- Human class I genes consist of the HLA-A, HLA-B, and HLA-C loci; associated gene products are found on all nucleated cells.
- The class II region genes consist of the D region, which is subdivided into HLA-DP, HLA-DQ, and HLA-DR subregions; the class II molecules are found on antigen-presenting cells.
- All MHC molecules show high allotypic polymorphism.

GENETICS

Codominant Gene Expression

Codominant expression of genes defined for pairs of heterozygous alleles leads to the situation in which both phenotypes may be present, or the expression of two alleles results in a blend of traits. For example, the codominantly expressed blood type AB is qualitatively distinct from either parental type A or B.

●●● STRUCTURE OF MHC CLASS I AND CLASS II MOLECULES

Each class I locus codes for a transmembrane polypeptide of molecular weight approximately 45 kDa, containing three extracellular domains (α_1, α_2, α_3). The molecule is expressed at the cell surface in a noncovalent association with an invariant polypeptide called β_2-microglobulin (β_2M) of 12 kDa. β_2M is a member of the Ig superfamily; the complex of class I and β_2M is expressed as a molecule with four domains associated such that the β_2M and α_3 domain of class I are juxtaposed near the cell surface membrane (Fig. 5-2).

Class II molecules have two transmembrane polypeptide chains (α and β, 30–34 and 26–29 kDa, respectively); the peptide-binding site is shared by the two domains farthest from the cell membrane. The overall structure of the peptide-binding site is very similar for both class I and class II MHC molecules; the base is made of β-pleated sheet, as in an immunoglobulin domain; the sides of the groove that holds the peptide are α-helices. Peptides bind within the allele-specific pockets defined by the two transmembrane polypeptide chains, where they are presented to the TCR for recognition. The extracellular domain shows variability in amino acid sequences, yielding grooves with different shapes. These grooves cradle the processed antigen for interaction with the T-cell receptor (Fig. 5-3). The class II MHC molecule is capable of presenting peptides of slightly larger size than that presented by the class I MHC complex.

Class I and class II genes also exhibit polymorphism with multiple allelic forms expressed. In humans, allelic forms are designated in descriptive manner. For examples, human class II genes are given numbers, such as HLA-D4 or HLA-D7, dependent upon loci location.

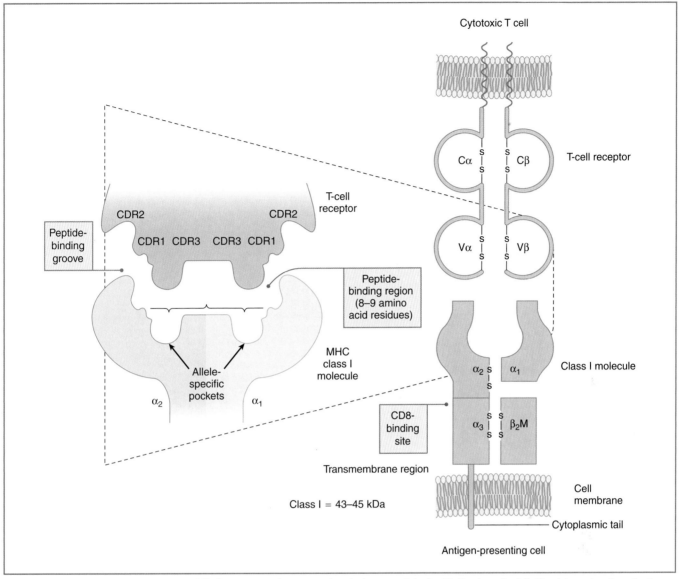

Figure 5-2. MHC class I. The class I MHC transmembrane molecule is associated with the invariant β_2M, giving structure to the extracellular domain for presentation of processed antigen to cytotoxic T cells. Interaction of the T-cell receptor is stabilized by CD8 recognition of the class I molecule. Shown here is a short peptide fragment (8–10 amino acids in length) noncovalently interacting with the α_1 and α_2 domains on the class I molecule and complementarity determining regions (CDRs) on the TCR.

KEY POINTS ABOUT STRUCTURE OF MHC CLASS I AND CLASS II MOLECULES

- Class I molecules are important in presentation of antigen epitopes to CD8$^+$ T cells. Each class I locus codes for a transmembrane polypeptide containing three extracellular domains (α_1, α_2, α_3), which is expressed at the cell surface in a noncovalent association with β_2-microglobulin (β_2M).

- Class II molecules present antigen to CD4$^+$ lymphocytes. Class II molecules have two transmembrane polypeptide chains. Peptides bind within the allele-specific pockets defined by the two transmembrane polypeptide chains, where they are presented to the TCR for recognition.

●●● MHC AND ANTIGEN PRESENTATION

Antigen is recognized by T cells when it is presented in complex with proteins of the major histocompatibility complex. Different antigen degradation and processing pathways produce MHC-peptide complexes in which endogenous (cytoplasmic) peptides associate with class I molecules and exogenous (endosomal) peptides associate with class II molecules. MHC class I presents endogenous Ag epitopes to CD8$^+$ T cytotoxic cells, and MHC class II presents exogenous Ag epitopes to CD4$^+$ T$_H$ cells. All nucleated cells are capable of presenting MHC class I, but only specialized phagocytic cells present antigenic epitopes on MHC class II.

Figure 5-3. MHC class II. Processed antigenic fragments (13–25 amino acids in length) interact with the α_1 and β_1 domains on the class II molecule within the peptide-binding groove, allowing presentation to CD4$^+$ T$_H$ cells. Interactions with the TCR are stabilized by CD4 recognition of conserved regions on the class II molecule.

Endogenous (Cytoplasmic) Antigen Processing and MHC Class I Presentation

MHC class I molecules bind peptide fragments derived from proteolytically degraded proteins endogenously synthesized by a cell (Fig. 5-4). Examples of endogenously produced antigens include proteins produced during intracellular viral replication. Small peptides are transported into the endoplasmic reticulum, where they associate with nascent MHC class I molecules before being routed through the Golgi apparatus and displayed on the surface for recognition by cytotoxic T lymphocytes. MHC class I molecules bind small antigenic peptides that are 8–10 amino acid residues in length. Upon recognition by CTLs, the CD8 molecule binds to constant domains on the class I a chain to stabilize the

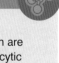

BIOCHEMISTRY

ATP-Mediated Intracellular Transporters

The transporters associated with antigen presentation are cytosolic proteases that shuttle peptides into the exocytic compartment for association with nascent MHC class I molecules. Specifically, TAP-1 and TAP-2 are members of the ATP-binding cassette transporter superfamily, which utilizes ATP to drive the transport of molecules across all cell membranes.

interaction. When T-cell (CTL) receptor binds antigen-MHC class I and costimulatory signals occur, the CTL is activated to produce and secrete toxin that kills the cell to which it is bound.

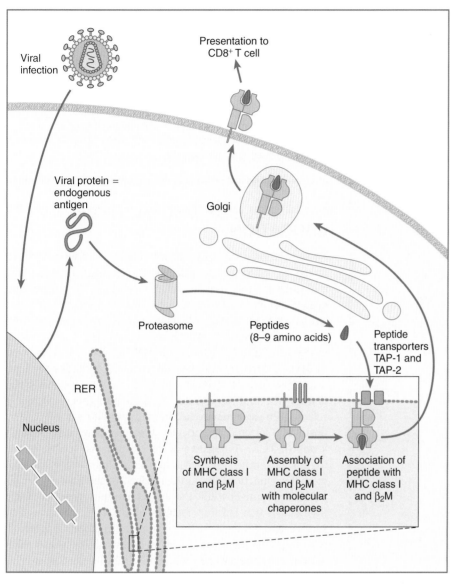

Figure 5-4. Endogenous pathway for antigen processing and class I presentation. Class I MHC molecules interact with peptides degraded by proteasomes, part of a large cytoplasmic proteolytic complex called the low-molecular-mass polypeptide (LMP). Degraded peptides are carried into the rough endoplasmic reticulum (RER) by transporters of antigenic peptides (TAP-1, TAP-2). Upon peptide binding, the interaction between a class I MHC α chain and β_2M is stabilized and the complex is routed through the Golgi to the plasma membrane.

Exogenous (Endosomal) Antigen Processing and MHC Class II Presentation

MHC class II molecules bind peptide fragments derived from proteolytically degraded proteins exogenously internalized by *antigen-presenting cells*, including macrophages, dendritic cells, and B cells (Fig. 5-5). Examples of exogenous antigens include degraded products resulting from phagocytosed bacterial agents. The resulting peptide fragments are compartmentalized in the endosome, where they associate with MHC class II molecules before being routed to the cell surface for recognition by helper T lymphocytes. MHC class II molecules bind larger antigenic peptides usually 13–25 amino acid residues in length (or longer).

Like class I molecules, class II MHC molecules are synthesized in the rough endoplasmic reticulum. The class II α and β chains reside there as a complex with an additional polypeptide called the invariant chain (Ii). The invariant chain blocks the groove of the class II molecule and prevents endogenous antigens from binding there. The MHC–invariant chain complex is transported to an acidic endosomal or lysosomal compartment that contains a degraded antigen peptide. The invariant chain comes off the complex, exposes the groove of the class II molecule, and allows the antigen peptide to slip into the groove. The class II antigen–peptide complex is then transported to the surface of the APC, where it is available for interaction with CD4+ T_H cells. When the CD4+ T-cell receptor binds antigen-MHC class II, and when appropriate costimulatory molecules are engaged, the CD4+ T cell is activated to proliferate and secrete cytokines, which in turn activate other cells of the immune system to generate humoral or cellular immunity.

B cells are excellent exogenous peptide presenter cells. The B cell can specifically phagocytose antigen via binding through surface immunoglobulin. Antigen is internalized, broken down to peptides presented on the B-cell surface in the peptide binding grooves of MHC class II molecules. The subsequent interaction of a B cell with a primed T cell that

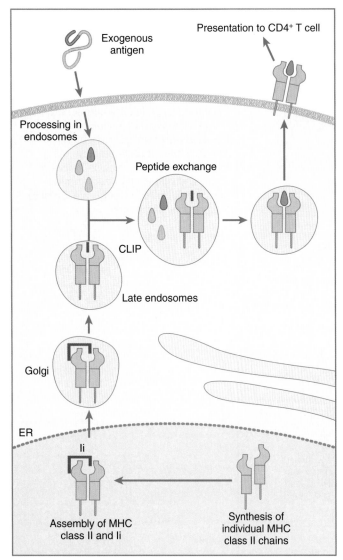

Figure 5-5. Exogenous pathway for antigen processing and class II presentation. The exogenous (endosomal) pathway prepares processed antigens for presentation to T cells via class II–regulated mechanisms. Nascent class II α and β polypeptides produced in the endoplasmic reticulum (ER) combine and interact with a specialized invariant chain (Ii) that prevents peptide binding within this intracellular compartment. The Ii fills the peptide-binding pocket and facilitates routing of the complex to the endosomal compartment. Late in the exogenous processing pathway, endosomes containing class II MHC molecules and the invariant chain fuse with lysosomes. Enzymes within the lysosomes degrade the invariant chain, enabling the class II MHC molecules to bind peptides.

recognizes the peptide–class II complex results in proliferative and activation pathways, which drive isotype switching as well as maturation of the B lymphocyte to become an antibody-secreting plasma cell. Importantly, since all nucleated cells express class I molecules, B cells have the innate ability to process antigen for incorporation of peptides into class I or class II presentation pathways.

KEY POINTS ABOUT MHC AND ANTIGEN PRESENTATION

- Different antigen degradation and processing pathways produce MHC–peptide complexes in which *endogenous* peptides associate with class I molecules and *exogenous* peptides associate with class II molecules.
- MHC class I molecules bind small antigenic peptides that are 8–10 amino acid residues in length; MHC class II molecules present slightly larger peptides.

●●● ROLE OF MHC IN THYMIC EDUCATION

The education process by which T cells in the thymus learn to recognize antigenic peptides in the context of self-MHC molecules is a two-step procedure involving both positive and negative selection. Immature T cells (thymocytes) interact with thymic epithelial cells that express high levels of both class I and class II MHC molecules. Thymocytes with moderate affinities for these self-MHC molecules are allowed to develop further, while thymocytes with affinities too high or too low for self-MHC are induced to die by apoptosis. The thymocytes that survive are said to have been *positively selected* through their weak interaction with self-MHC. The positively selected thymocytes then begin to express high levels of TCR. A negative selection process occurs as the thymocytes travel deeper into the cortex, at the cortico-medullary junction, and in the medulla of the thymus. At this point, self-antigens fill the MHC peptide grooves. Only thymocytes that fail to recognize self-antigens are allowed to survive and proceed further along the maturation process, with the remainder undergoing apoptosis. This ensures elimination of self-reactive T cells. Eventually, T cells that survive the negative selection process lose either CD4 or CD8, becoming *single positive* cells. Fewer than 5% of thymocytes survive selection and leave the thymus to take up residence in the secondary lymphoid organs.

KEY POINT ABOUT THE ROLE OF MHC IN THYMIC EDUCATION

- T cells in the thymus learn to recognize "foreign" antigenic peptides in the context of self-MHC molecules by a two-step process involving both positive and negative selection.

●●● ROLE OF MHC IN ACTIVATION OF T CELLS

Binding between the TCR and the MHC–antigen peptide complex is highly specific and acts as the first signal to induce T-cell activation. Mature T cells do not respond to either self-MHC alone or to free peptide. Activated T cells differ from resting T cells in that they proliferate and secrete lymphokines or lytic substances. The affinity of the TCR for the

MHC–antigen complex often is too low to fully activate the T cell; in addition to interactions with CD4 or CD8, numerous accessory molecules increase avidity between the T cell and APC by performing both adhesive and costimulatory signaling functions (Fig. 5-6).

●●● ASSOCIATION OF DISEASE WITH MHC HAPLOTYPE

Particular MHC alleles are associated with better protection against certain infections, while others have been identified as associated with a greater chance of developing autoimmunity. Some diseases are distinctly more common in individuals with a particular MHC allele or MHC haplotype. Diseases with a strong association with certain MHC alleles include insulin-dependent diabetes mellitus and Graves' disease. For example, expression of HLA-DR4 is associated with rheumatoid arthritis. Nearly 90% of people with ankylosing spondylitis carry the HLA-B27 allele. Expression of HLA-DR2 is associated with multiple sclerosis. It is hypothesized that in some cases MHC molecules serve as receptors for the attachment and entry of pathogens into the cell; this makes individuals with a certain HLA type more susceptible to infection by a particular intracellular pathogen using that HLA molecule as a receptor. Alternatively, an infectious agent might possess antigenic determinants that resemble MHC molecules (molecular mimicry). Such resemblance might allow the pathogen to escape immune detection because it is seen as *self*, or it may induce an autoimmune reaction. Because MHC molecules differ in their ability to accommodate different peptides, individuals who express certain MHC genes may lack the ability to present microbial epitopes capable of inducing protective T-cell responses. Finally, there may simply be no T cells capable of recognizing a particular MHC–antigen combination, leading to a "hole in the T-cell repertoire."

KEY POINTS ABOUT THE ASSOCIATION OF DISEASE WITH MHC HAPLOTYPE

- Certain MHC alleles are associated with a greater chance of protective immune responses to pathogens, as well as toward developing autoimmunity.

- Some diseases are distinctly more common in individuals with a particular MHC allele or MHC haplotype.

Figure 5-6. Accessory molecules involved in antigen presentation. The binding between the MHC–antigen peptide complex and the TCR acts as the first signal toward induction of T-cell activation. Accessory molecules increase avidity between T cell and APC by performing additional adhesive and signaling functions. Adhesion molecules, such as LFA-1 (CD11a/CD18; leukocyte function–associated antigen–1) and ICAM-1 (CD54; intracellular adhesion molecule–1) pairing, promote firm adhesion between T cell and APC and can provide costimulatory signals for T-cell activation. This interaction also facilitates T-cell sampling of antigen in the context of MHC molecules on the surface of the APC. Additionally, T cells require further costimulation through binding of CD28 with either of its ligands, CD80 or CD86 (B7.1 or B7.2). If all events transpire, full activation of the T cell occurs, leading to production of T-cell cytokines and a proliferative response.

●●● ATYPICAL AND UNIQUE ANTIGEN PRESENTATION

Superantigens Directly Bind T-Cell Receptors and MHC Without Processing

Superantigens are defined by their ability to stimulate a large fraction of T cells via interaction with the T-cell receptor Vβ domain (Fig. 5-7). Superantigens are predominantly bacterial in origin, such as staphylococcal enterotoxin and toxin-1 responsible for toxic shock syndrome. The superantigen circumvents normal processing and directly bridges the TCR

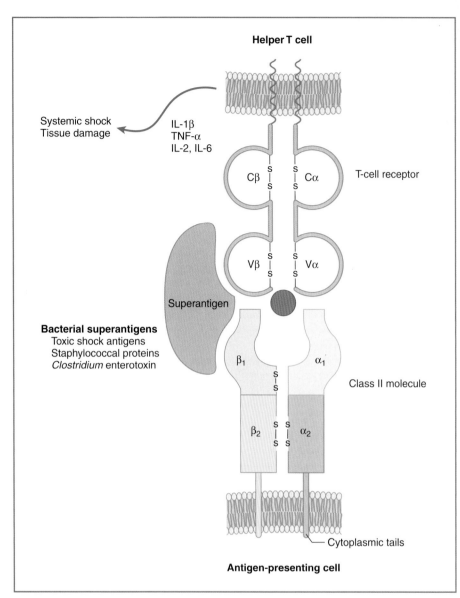

Figure 5-7. Superantigens. T cells of various antigenic specificities are activated when bacterial superantigens cross-link MHC class II molecules with common TCR Vβ regions. All T cells that express that particular Vβ region are subject to activation, causing massive release of cytokines and subsequent symptoms of shock and host injury. This occurs regardless of antigen specificity and the peptide that fills the MHC class II groove.

with the MHC class II molecule, causing cells to divide and differentiate into effector cells and release T-cell factors (IL-2, TNF-α, and IL-1β). Because the number of T cells that share Vβ domains is high (up to 10% of all T cells), large numbers of T cells (regardless of antigen specificity) may be activated by superantigens. This can lead to massive systemic disruption with symptoms similar to septic shock including occurrence of severe tissue injury and possible multiple organ failure.

Presentation of Nonclassical Lipid Antigens to T Cells

The CD1 molecules represent a novel lineage of antigen-presenting molecules. They are distinct from MHC classes I and II; the CD1 family of non-MHC locus-encoded proteins present nonpeptide glycolipid antigens to T cells (Fig. 5-8). In humans, there are five distinct CD1 proteins (CD1a, b, c, d, and e). The CD1 molecules have similar structure to MHC

class I, with three extracellular domains and a noncovalently associated β₂-microglobulin. The peptide groove is lined with nonpolar/hydrophobic side chains in which antigen binds in a deep, narrow hydrophobic pocket; ligands interact via hydrophobic interactions rather than by hydrogen bonding. Although the role of the CD1 in pathogenesis has not been determined, it is an area of active investigation.

KEY POINTS ABOUT ATYPICAL AND UNIQUE ANTIGEN PRESENTATION

- Superantigens cross-link T-cell receptors and MHC independent of antigen and antigen processing, usually via direct interaction with the TCR Vβ region.
- The CD1 family of non-MHC locus-encoded proteins presents nonpeptide glycolipid antigens to T cells.

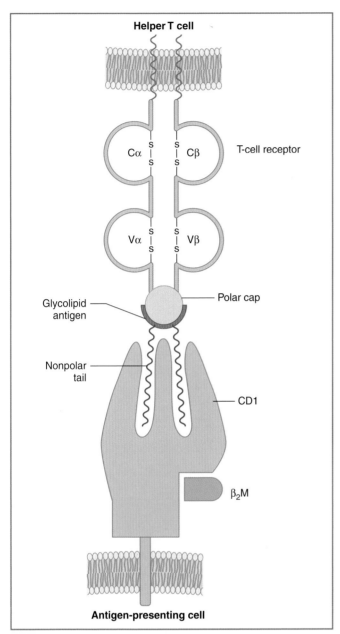

Figure 5-8. Nonclassical lipid antigen presentation by CD1 molecules. The peptide groove of the CD1 surface molecule is lined with nonpolar, hydrophobic side chains. The CD1 molecule binds antigen in a deep, narrow hydrophobic pocket, enabling presentation to the T-cell receptor.

Innate Immunity

6

The innate immune system is composed of components present prior to manifestation of infection. These components include physical defensive barriers as well as factors that recognize classes of molecules frequently encountered on invading pathogens. Innate defensive measures allow containment of organisms while the specific immune response is either generated or up-regulated.

●●● PHYSICAL BARRIERS AGAINST INFECTION

Four major categories of physical barriers exist to limit entry and control expansion of foreign pathogens. Defensive roles may be *anatomic* (skin, mucous membranes), *physiologic* (temperature, low pH, chemical mediators), *phagocytic* (digestion of microorganisms), or *inflammatory* (vascular fluid leakage).

Anatomic Barrier

The skin and mucous membranes provide an effective barrier against microorganisms. The skin has the thin outer epidermis and the thicker underlying dermis to impede entry, as well as sebaceous glands to produce sebum. Sebum is made of lactic acid and fatty acids, which effectively reduce skin pH to between 3 and 5 to inhibit organism growth. Mucous membranes are covered by cilia, which trap organisms in mucus and propel them out of the body.

Physiologic Barrier

The physiologic barrier includes factors such as temperature, low pH, and chemical mediators. Many organisms cannot survive or multiply in elevated body temperature. Soluble proteins such as lysozymes, interferons, and complement components play a major role in innate immunity. Lysozymes can interact with bacterial cell walls; interferons alpha and beta are natural inhibitors of viral growth; complement components use both specific and nonspecific immune factors to convert inactive forms to active moieties that damage membranes of pathogens. Low pH in the stomach and gastric environment discourages bacterial growth.

Phagocytic and Endocytic Barriers

Blood monocytes, tissue macrophages, and neutrophils phagocytose and kill microorganisms via multiple complex digestion mechanisms. Bacteria become attached to cell membranes and are ingested into phagocytic vesicles. Phagosomes fuse with lysosomes where lysosomal enzymes digest captured organisms.

HISTOLOGY

The Skin

The skin is composed of a thin outer epidermis and thicker underlying dermis and assists in impeding entry of foreign organisms. The interface between the two tissues is demarcated by epidermal ridges and dermal papillae, with interpapillary pegs dividing ridges. Production of sebum (lactic acid and fatty acids) through short ducts emanating from sebaceous glands effectively reduces skin pH, which inhibits the growth of microorganisms.

Inflammatory Barriers

Invading organisms cause localized tissue damage leading to complex inflammatory responses (Fig. 6-1). Initial damage and entry of organisms result in release of chemotactic factors (complement components, chemokines, fibrinopeptides) to signal changes in nearby vasculature, allowing extravasation of polymorphonuclear cells to the injury site. Celsus (first century AD) described the four cardinal signs of inflammation as *rubor* (redness), *tumor* (swelling), *calor* (heat), and *dolor* (pain). Later, Galen (second century AD) added a fifth sign: *functio laesa* (loss of function).

PATHOLOGY

Acute Respiratory Distress Syndrome (ARDS)

ARDS is characterized by lung inflammation caused by excessive nitric oxide and inflammatory cascades, leading ultimately to vasodilatation and fluid exudation. Congestion of the vessels and proteinaceous acellular edema occur in the alveoli with accumulation of vividly eosinophilic, acellular hyaline membranes against alveolar septae.

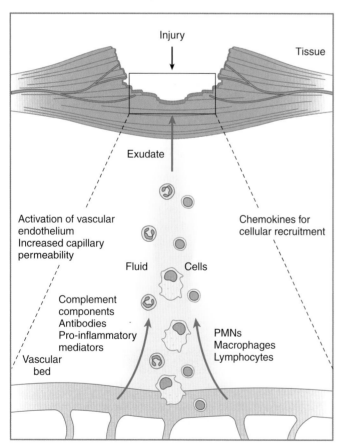

Figure 6-1. Inflammatory response. Inflammatory responses lead to vasodilation, causing erythema (redness) and increased temperature, and increased capillary permeability, which allows exudates (fluid) to accumulate, leading to tissue swelling (edema) and influx of cells to site of tissue damage. Once cells enter the area of injury, they release chemotactic factors to recruit additional cells, leading to local activation at the damaged site.

KEY POINTS ABOUT PHYSICAL BARRIERS

- Innate defense barriers include (1) anatomic barriers, (2) physiologic barriers, (3) phagocytic barriers, and (4) inflammatory barriers.
- Damage to tissue caused by invading pathogens can lead to *rubor, tumor, calor, dolor,* and *functio laesa.*
- Tissue damage leads to an influx of inflammatory cells through chemotaxis, activation, margination, and diapedesis.

●●● DEFENSIVE INNATE RESPONDING CELLS

The cell types involved in innate immune responses include the polymorphonuclear cells (primarily neutrophils), monocytes and macrophages, eosinophils, and natural killer (NK) cells. Some of these cells are capable of killing target cells via nonspecific (nonantigen/MHC-dependent) means through release of lytic enzymes, perforin, or tumor necrosis factor (TNF). Others are involved in phagocytic mechanisms that kill via intracellular processes.

Neutrophils

Neutrophils are typically the first infiltrating cell type to the site of inflammation (Fig. 6-2). Activated endothelial cells increase expression of E-selectin and P-selectin, which are recognized by neutrophil surface mucins (PSGL-1 or sialyl Lewis[x] on glycoproteins or glycolipids), and induce neutrophil rolling along the endothelium. Chemoattractants (e.g., IL-8) can trigger firm adhesion and diapedesis. Subsequent chemotaxis is further induced by IL-8, along with multiple complement components (e.g., C5a), fibrinopeptides, and leukotrienes. Activated neutrophils express high-affinity Fc receptors and complement receptors to allow increased phagocytosis of invading organisms. Activation of neutrophils leads to the respiratory burst, producing reactive oxygen and nitrogen intermediates as well as release of primary and secondary granules containing proteases, phospholipases, elastases, and collagenases. Pus, a yellowish white, opaque creamy matter produced by the process of suppuration, consists of innumerable neutrophils (some dead and dying) and tissue debris.

Mononuclear Cells and Macrophages

Macrophages involved in innate immunity include *alveolar macrophages* in the lung, *histocytes* in connective tissue, *Kupffer cells* in liver, *mesangial cells* in kidney, *microglial cells* in brain, and *osteoclasts* in bone. Chemokine mediators such as macrophage inflammatory protein-1α (MIP-1α) and MIP-1β attract monocytes to the site of pathogenic infection (Table 6-1). Like the neutrophil, monocytes express surface ligands (e.g., integrin a4b1, also called VLA-4) that recognize ligands (e.g., vascular cell adhesion molecule-1 [VCAM-1])

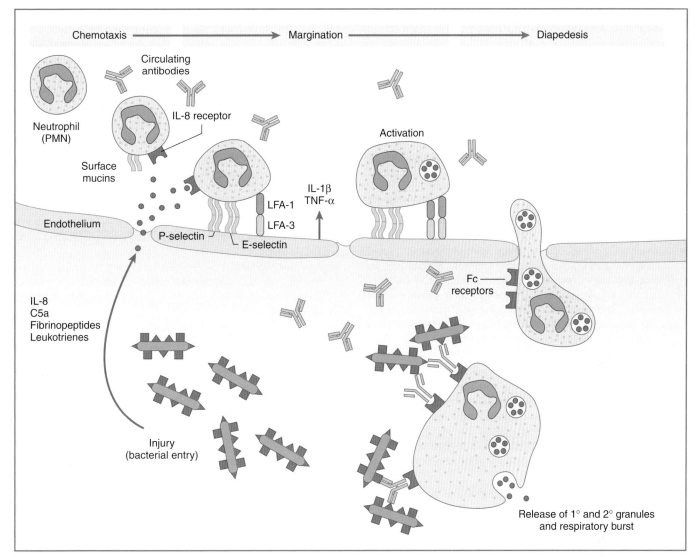

Figure 6-2. Events associated with neutrophil transendothelial migration. Bacteria entering through a breach in the mechanical barrier (skin) trigger release of chemotactic factors that up-regulate selectins on endothelial beds. Circulating polymorphonuclear cells interact via weak binding surface mucins; interactions are enhanced in the presence of stimulating factors (IL-1, IL-8, TNF-α), leading to further cellular activation, margination, and diapedesis. Pictured are neutrophils, which when entering tissue undergo respiratory burst and release of primary and secondary granules upon cross-linking of Fc receptors to antibodies recognizing bacterial epitopes.

TABLE 6-1. Partial List of Chemokines Produced by Monocytes and Macrophages

Chemokine Class*	Chemokine	Cells Affected
CC	MIP-1α	Monocytes, NK cells, T cells, dendritic cells
	MIP-1β	Monocytes, NK cells, T cells, dendritic cells
	MCP-1	Monocytes, NK cells, T cells, dendritic cells
	Eotaxin	T cells, eosinophils
CXC	IL-8	Neutrophils, (naïve T cells)
	GROα, β, γ	Neutrophils, (naïve T cells)
	IP-10	Monocytes, NK cells, T cells

*In general, chemokines fall mainly into two distinct groups. The *CC chemokines* have two adjacent cysteine residues (hence the name "CC"). The *CXC chemokines* have an amino acid between two cysteine residues. Monocytes and macrophages produce small polypeptides that are chemotactic for leukocytes, acting through receptors that are members of the G-protein coupled signal transducing family. All chemokines are related in amino acid sequence and their receptors are integral membrane proteins that are characterized by containing seven membrane-spanning helices. Each chemokine reacts with one or more receptors and can affect multiple cell types.

on endothelial cells. This interaction can mediate cell rolling, firm adhesion, and diapedesis. Activated tissue macrophages secrete proinflammatory mediators in response to bacteria and bacterial products, including IL-1, IL-6, IL-8, IL-12, and TNF-α. TNF-α is an inducer of a local inflammatory response that helps contain infections. IL-8 also is involved in the local inflammatory response, helping attract neutrophils to the site of infection. IL-1, IL-6, and TNF-α have a critical role in inducing the acute-phase response in the liver and inducing fever, which limits bacterial growth and upregulates host defense in several ways. IL-12 may also activate NK cells.

KEY POINTS ABOUT DEFENSIVE INNATE RESPONDING CELLS

- Immune responses of the innate immune system provide natural immunity against microorganisms via phagocytosis and intracellular killing, recruitment of other inflammatory cells, and presentation of antigens. Leukocytes that provide innate immunity are derived from *myeloid* lineage. These cells include highly phagocytic, motile neutrophils, monocytes and tissue macrophages, eosinophils, and natural killer (NK) cells. These cells provide the first line of defense against most pathogens.

- Neutrophils are usually the first cell type to arrive at the site of tissue damage. Activation leads to respiratory bursts and release of granules to control bacterial growth. Mononuclear cells and macrophages engulf organisms via multiple mechanisms, leading to control and destruction within intracellular phagosomes. NK cells are large granular lymphocytes that kill targets via ADCC or through lysis using either Fas-mediated or perforin-induced mechanisms.

- Chemokines and complement components are critical for activation of innate immune functions. Defects may lead to severe clinical complications.

●●● MICROBIAL AGENT RECOGNITION THROUGH PATTERN-RECOGNITION RECEPTORS

Monocytes and macrophages express receptors that recognize broad structural motifs highly conserved within microbial species. Such receptors are referred to as pattern-recognition receptors (PRRs). Engagement of these receptors leads to immediate triggering of signal pathways that promote phagocytosis (Fig. 6-3), an event that requires actin and myosin polymerization. Multiple factors assist in preparing the particulate for engulfment and targeting for destruction, including various opsonins composed of complement components. Examples of these include receptors that recognize common bacterial carbohydrate elements, such as LPS, mannose, and glucans (glycogen polysaccharides). A unique family of membrane-bound receptors, termed the Toll-like receptors (TLRs), plays a critical role in recognition of bacterial components (cell wall membranes, LPS, flagellin, CpG oligodeoxynucleotides); interaction with any of these receptors initiates proinflammatory responses that function locally and systemically.

The process of phagocytosis compartmentalizes the invading pathogen into an intracellular vacuole referred to as a *phagosome*. The phagosome fuses with intracellular lysosomes, forming a phagolysosome vacuole. The lysosome is extremely acidic in nature and contains powerful lytic enzymes; fusion with the phagosome allows directed delivery for targeted destruction of invading organisms. In addition, phagocytosis triggers a mechanism known as the *respiratory burst*, leading to production of toxic metabolites that assist in the killing process. The most critical of these toxic metabolites are nitric oxide, hydrogen peroxides, and superoxide anions.

KEY POINT ABOUT MICROBIAL AGENT RECOGNITION THROUGH PATTERN-RECOGNITION RECEPTORS

- Pattern-recognition receptors (PRRs) present on innate immune system cells assist in the recognition of bacteria and virions. Recognition by PRRs leads to activation of multiple facets of cellular response.

●●● LINKING INNATE AND ADAPTIVE IMMUNE RESPONSES

Phagocytosed or pinocytosed antigens processed by APCs may then be presented to the adaptive immune system cells. Dendritic cells, macrophages and monocytes, and B cells are extremely good at presenting antigens to T lymphocytes. The context in which the T cell recognizes antigen, the abundance of antigen, and the duration of antigen exposure are important parameters that affect the nature and maturation of the T-cell response. The most effective activators of T cells are mature, activated dendritic cells (DCs). These dendritic populations have a high expression of MHC and costimulatory molecules, which are required for maximal T-cell stimulation (Fig. 6-4).

HISTOLOGY

Cytoskeletal Remodeling During Phagocytosis

The cellular cytoskeleton exists as a three-dimensional network of fibrils to form a supporting scaffold to anchor structures to the plasma membrane or membrane-bound proteins, or to serve as "tracks" for organelle intracellular movement. Phagocytosis of microorganisms involves remodeling of the macrophage cytoskeleton, with regulated changes to lamellipodia. Receptor-mediated endocytosis involves engulfment of particulates with fission into membrane-bound vesicles via clathrin-coated pits; vesicle membranes are recycled to the plasma membrane, while the internalized materials are delivered to lysosomal compartments.

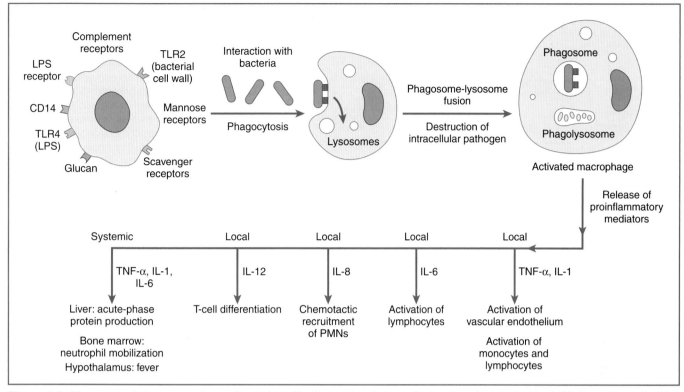

Figure 6-3. Phagocytosis by macrophages leads to activation and pathogen destruction. IL, interleukin; LPS, lipopolysaccharide; PMN, polymorphonuclear cell; TLR, Toll-like receptor.

●●● NATURAL KILLER CELLS: EARLY DEFENDERS AGAINST INFECTION

NK cells are large granular lymphocytes that nonspecifically kill virus-infected cells and tumor cells. NK cells share many surface molecules with T lymphocytes. Killing by NK cells is enhanced by cytokines such as IFN-α, IFN-β and IL-12, and further activation can occur in the presence of activated T cells. NK cells may be activated by microorganisms to produce cytokines (IL-2, IFN-γ, IFN-α, and TNF-α). These circulating large granular lymphocytes do not express CD3, TCR, or immunoglobulin but display surface receptors (CD16) for the Fc fragment of IgG antibodies. The NK cells are able to kill "self" in the absence of antigen-specific receptors. They can also kill by means of *antibody-dependent cell-mediated cytotoxicity* (ADCC) mechanisms via their Fc receptors (Fig. 6-5). NK cells mediate lysis target cells by release of lytic granules and perforin-induced pore formation.

Additionally, NK cells can kill target cells using Fas/Fas-ligand (FasL)–mediated apoptotic pathways. NK cells bear FasL on their surface and can kill Fas-bearing target cells. NK cells do not express specific antigen receptors. Rather, NK cells use two categories of receptors to deliver either activation or inhibition signals. These opposing signals mediate activity. Activation receptors (carbohydrate-binding proteins) are always present on the surface of NK cells. Engagement of inhibitory signals (KIR and/or CD94) on the surface of the NK cell with class I MHC on the target cell counteracts activation. During viral infection, the level of class I MHC decreases on the infected target, thus allowing NK cells to be fully activated to destroy the target cell.

●●● COMPLEMENT IN INFLAMMATION AND IMMUNITY

Complement is a system of more than 30 serum and cell-surface proteins involved in inflammation and immunity. In conjunction with specific antibodies, complement components act as the primary humoral defense system against bacterial and viral infections. Most of the complement proteins in the serum are produced by liver hepatocytes. Some of the complement components are acute-phase proteins and can increase in concentration by two- to three-fold. Many of the complement proteins have shared sequences, indicating that they evolved by gene duplication and recombination.

Complement Cascades

Complement activation involves the sequential activation of complement proteins, either by protein-protein interactions or by proteolytic cleavage. At each step, the number of protein molecules activated increases, amplifying the reaction. Many complement proteins are present as *zymogens* (inactive precursors), which are activated either by conformational changes or by proteolytic cleavage by other complement proteins. Activation of these zymogens results in specific serine protease activity capable of cleaving other

Figure 6-4. Link between innate and adaptive (acquired) immunity. Pathogen recognition through pattern-recognition receptors is an important bridge between innate and adaptive immune function. Recognition leads to activation and maturation of the presenting cell. Processed antigen is presented to naïve T cells, accompanied by secretion of cytokines to assist development and maturation of T-cell phenotypic response (e.g., T_H1 maturation via presence of IL-12). Inset box shows important Toll-like receptors and specific ligands involved in pathogen recognition.

Toll-like receptor	Ligand
TLR1, 2, 6	Gram-positive LPS
TLR3	dsRNA
TLR4	Gram-negative LPS
TLR5	Flagellin
TLR9	Unmethylated CpG DNA

complement proteins, producing the complement cascade. Three pathways are described for complement activation. The *classical pathway* is initiated by the presence of antigen-antibody complexes. The *alternative pathway* is initiated by recognition of foreign cell surfaces. The *lectin pathway* (or *mannose-binding pathway*) recognizes mannose on pathogenic organisms (Fig. 6-6).

The classical complement pathway is initiated by immuno-complexes of antigen and antibody. Complement factor C1 (composed of C1q, C1r, and C1s) is activated through requisite cross-linking of two antibodies through Fc region binding. Alternatively, one pentameric IgM molecule may serve as the catalyst. Activated C1 complex can catalyze the cleavage of C4, followed by C2, yielding C4b2b, which is known as the C3 convertase. The C3 convertase amplifies breakdown of C3 into C3a and C3b; C3a is a powerful chemotactic factor that can also increase vascular permeability. C3b joins with the C4b2b complex to form the C5 convertase. Breakdown of C5 leads to production of C5a, another powerful chemotactic factor and macrophage activator. C5b forms the basis for creation of the membrane

attack complex (MAC), which in essence assembles pore structures within cell membranes, leading to hypotonic lysis of target cells. Whereas the small C5a fragment is released into the blood as a potent complement anaphylatoxin, the large C5b molecule binds proteins C6 and C7. The complex C5b67 has hydrophobic regions that permit it to insert into the lipid bilayer of nearby cell membranes. Subsequent binding of C8 permits some leakage of cell contents, causing slow lysis. This process is accelerated by binding of multiple C9 molecules, which assemble to form a protein channel through the membrane. C9 is analogous to perforins produced by cytolytic T cells and NK cells. C5b6789 thereby forms the basis of the MAC; the MAC is especially critical for elimination of bacteria resistant to intracellular killing by phagocytes.

The classical pathway of complement can also be activated by a serum mannose-binding lectin (MBL) complex. This complex is structurally similar to the C1 complex. However, instead of binding to immunocomplexes, it binds directly to polysaccharides on gram-negative bacteria. The MBL is C1q-like in structure, and the mannose-associated serine proteases

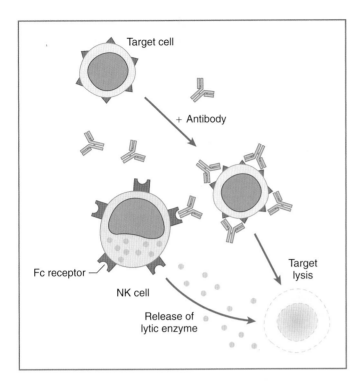

Figure 6-5. Antibody-dependent cell-mediated cytotoxicity (ADCC). ADCC is a phenomenon by which target cells coated with antibody are destroyed by specialized killer cells. Among the cells that mediate ADCC are NK cells, neutrophils, and eosinophils. The killing cells express receptors for the Fc portion of antibodies that coat targets. Recognition of antibody-coated targets leads to release of lytic enzymes at the site of Fc-mediated contact. Target cell killing may also involve perforin-mediated membrane damage. Eosinophils can function in a similar manner to kill large parasites.

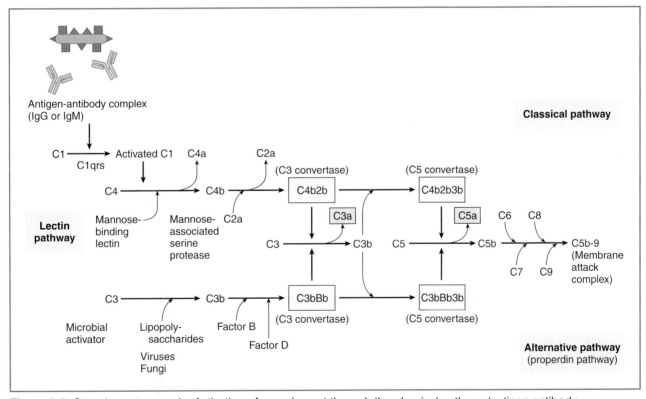

Figure 6-6. Complement cascade. Activation of complement through the *classical pathway* (antigen-antibody complexes), the *alternative pathway* (recognition of foreign cell surfaces), or the *lectin pathway* (or *mannose-binding pathway*) promotes activation of C3 and C5, leading to construction of the membrane attack complex.

(MASPs) are similar to C1r and C1s. Upon binding bacterial surfaces, MBL-MASP can cleave C4 and C2 and thereby activate the remainder of the classical pathway.

The complement component C3 is the starting point for the alternative pathway. Cleavage of C3 exposes a reactive thioester bond that enables C3b to bind to bacterial cell surfaces. Factor B is bound, and the complex is cleaved by factor D, resulting in a C3bBb complex (called the C3 convertase). The *C3 convertase* allows amplification of enzymatic cleavage of C3 into more C3a and C3b. Factor H displaces B from C3bBb and further assists in the conversion of C3b to iC3b by acting as a cofactor for factor I. C3a can also bind to mast cells to cause release of histamines. iC3b acts to activate neutrophils and macrophages via CR3 receptors (in the absence of antibody).

Biological Functions of Complement

Activation of the complement system results in the production of several different polypeptide cleavage fragments that are involved in five primary biological functions of inflammation and immunity (Fig. 6-7).

Direct Cytolysis of Foreign Organisms

Antibodies recognizing pathogenic determinants form the basis of a physical structure with which complement components interact. Specifically, complement component C1 interacts with the Fc portion of IgM and IgG (except IgG4), binding to the surface of bacteria. The binding of C1 initiates a cascade of events whereby a MAC is built upon the cellular surface. Synthesis of the MAC structure culminates in assembly of a pore channel in the lipid bilayer, causing osmotic lysis of the cell. MAC formation requires prior activation by either the classical or the alternative pathway and utilizes the proteins C5b, C6, C7, C8, and C9.

Opsonization of Foreign Organisms

Complement components (e.g., C3b or inactivated C3b; iC3b) bind to pathogens. Interaction with receptors (CR1, CR2, CR3, and CR4) on the surface of macrophages, monocytes, and neutrophils leads to enhanced phagocytosis and targeted destruction of organisms.

Activation and Directed Migration of Leukocytes

Proteolytic degradation of C3 and C5 leads to production of leukocyte chemotactic factors referred to as anaphylatoxins.

For example, C3a is chemotactic for eosinophils. C5a is a much more potent chemokine, attracting neutrophils, monocytes and macrophages, and eosinophils. Interaction of C3a, C4a, or C5a with mast cells and basophils leads to release of histamine, serotonin, and other vasoactive amines, resulting in increased vascular permeability, causing inflammation and smooth muscle contraction.

Solubilization and Clearance of Immunocomplexes

One of the major roles complement plays is the solubilization and clearance of immunocomplexes from the circulation. First, C3b and C4b can covalently bind to the Fc region of insoluble immunocomplexes, disrupting the lattice and making them soluble. C3b and C4b bound to the immunocomplex are recognized by the CR1 receptor on erythrocytes, facilitating their transport to the liver and spleen. In the liver and spleen, the immunocomplexes are removed and phagocytosed by macrophage-like cells. The RBCs are returned to the circulation.

Enhancement of Humoral Immune Response

Coating of antigens with C3d (a breakdown product of C3) facilitates their delivery to germinal centers rich in B cells and follicular dendritic cells.

KEY POINTS ABOUT COMPLEMENT IN INFLAMMATION AND IMMUNITY

- The activities of complement include (1) cytolysis of foreign organisms, (2) opsonization and phagocytosis of foreign organisms, (3) activation of inflammation and directed migration of leukocytes, (4) solubilization and clearance of immunocomplexes, and (5) enhancement of humoral immune response.

- Complement activation results in the release of anaphylatoxins (C3a, C4a, and C5a). These are important mediators of inflammation, causing recruitment and activation of neutrophils, macrophages, and other cell types.

- Activation also produces cleavage products (C3b, C3bi, and C4b), which serve as opsonins, enhancing phagocytosis.

Figure 6-7. Biological functions of complement.

Adaptive Immune Response and Hypersensitivity

7

●●● T CELLS: PRIMARY EFFECTORS FOR CELL-MEDIATED IMMUNITY

The T cell is the primary effector for control and regulation of adaptive immune function. T helper 1 (T_H1) cells aid in the regulation of cellular immunity. T helper 2 (T_H2) cells aid B cells in isotype switching and in production of antibodies. Cytotoxic T cells (CTLs) mediate antigen-specific, major histocompatibility complex (MHC)–restricted cytotoxicity and are important for killing intracytoplasmic pathogens that are not accessible to secreted antibody or to phagocytes.

KEY POINTS ABOUT T CELLS
- Adaptive immune responses are mediated by effector lymphocytes.
- T_H cells provide assistance in regulation of cellular immunity and help to B cells for isotype switching and production of antibodies.
- Cytotoxic T cells (CTLs) mediate antigen-specific, MHC class I–restricted cytotoxicity and killing of intracellular pathogens.

●●● DEVELOPMENT OF T_H1 AND T_H2 PHENOTYPES

The development of T_H1 and T_H2 cellular phenotypes (defined primarily by patterns of cytokine expression) is under the control of local cytokines and factors (Fig. 7-1). Development of precursor T cells into the T_H1 phenotype gives rise to cells that promote cytotoxic and delayed-type hypersensitivity reactions as well as activate macrophages for increased protection against intracellular pathogens. The T_H1 cells are primarily characterized by secretion of IFN-γ and IL-2. T_H2 cells primarily secrete IL-4, IL-5, IL-6, and IL-10 and activate B cells for antibody production. Each phenotype produces cytokines that inhibit development of the alternate set; IFN-γ inhibits T_H2 development while IL-4 and IL-10 inhibit T_H1 development. In addition, precursor cells exhibit specific production of transcription factors (STAT4 or STAT6 and GATA3) that influence lineage development.

KEY POINTS ABOUT THE DEVELOPMENT OF T_H1 AND T_H2 PHENOTYPES
- The development of T_H response is dictated by local production of cytokines, giving rise to T_H1 or T_H2 cells from naïve precursor cells.
- Each subset produces a unique set of cytokine mediators, some of which inhibit development of the other phenotype.

●●● ROLE OF T CELLS IN B-CELL ACTIVATION

B cells are capable of presenting antigen, thus allowing direct elicitation of cytokines from T cells for stimulation, resulting in activation and plasma cell development (Fig. 7-2). Clonal expansion of B cells under the influence of T-cell cytokines leads to plasma cell development, isotype class switching, and production of memory responses. Specifically, IL-4 secreted from T_H2 cells acts as a B-cell growth factor, and IL-6 assists in delivering signals for maturation of the antibody response. Under certain circumstances, B cells can also respond and proliferate through T-independent mechanisms, usually

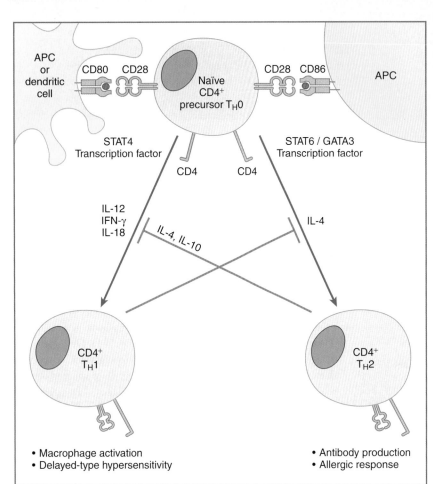

Figure 7-1. Development of T helper cell phenotypes. T_H1 and T_H2 cells derive from precursor cells (T_H0) under the influence of local cytokines. Each secretes a phenotypic subset of cytokines that drive effector responses. In addition, secreted cytokines modulate response to the other subset and inhibit alternative functional development.

involving antigens with long repeating epitopes that allow cross-linking of immunoglobulin receptors on the surface of the B cell. A common example of this occurs with bacterial capsid antigens containing repeating carbohydrate (polysaccharide) epitopes. In the case of T-independent activation, there is no accompanying maturation of response and antibody production is primarily limited to IgM production.

●●● DEVELOPMENT OF CYTOTOXIC T-CELL EFFECTORS

The CD8+ cytotoxic T cell recognizes antigen presented via class I MHC molecules. These require strong costimulatory signals to become effector cells (Fig. 7-3). CD8+ T cells can be activated by peptides presented by dendritic cells, which deliver a strong costimulatory signal through surface expression of molecules such as CD80 and CD86, which bind T-cell CD28, and intercellular adhesion molecule-1 (ICAM, CD54), which binds the T-cell integrin CD11a/CD18. Other APCs do not produce strong enough costimulatory signals; IL-2 from nearby CD4+ T_H1 cells recognizing peptide presented by class II MHC on the same APC is required to fully activate these CD8+ CTLs to become cytotoxic effectors.

●●● HYPERSENSITIVITY: INAPPROPRIATE RESPONSE RESULTING IN DISEASE

Hypersensitivity is a definable immune response that leads to deleterious host reactions rather than protection against disease. The hypersensitivity reactions fall into four classes based on their mechanisms and the ability to passively transfer response through antibodies or through T lymphocytes. These responses include inappropriate antigenic response, excessive magnitude of response, prolonged duration of response, and innocent bystander effect reactions leading to tissue damage.

Type I Hypersensitivity: IgE-Mediated Immediate Hypersensitivity

Type I hypersensitivity (also called *immediate hypersensitivity*) is due to aberrant production and activity of IgE against normally nonpathogenic antigens (commonly called *allergens*) (Fig. 7-4). The IgE binds to mast cells or basophils via high-affinity IgE receptors. Subsequent antigen exposure results in cross-linking of cell-bound IgE with activation

Figure 7-2. B-cell response to T-dependent and T-independent antigens. T_H2 cells specifically recognize class II–presented antigenic determinants and drive B-cell activation, leading to isotype class switching and antibody secretion (*left*). Alternatively, T-independent responses to repeating carbohydrate epitopes stimulate antibody production but do not lead to maturation of the antibody response.

(degranulation) of mast cells or basophils to release preformed mediators (e.g., vasoactive amines, histamine, leukotrienes, prostaglandin D_2) and to synthesize new mediators (i.e., chemotaxins, cytokines). These mediators are responsible for the signs and symptoms of allergic diseases. In severe cases, anaphylactic shock may occur, characterized by a sudden and sharp drop in blood pressure, urticaria, and breathing difficulties caused by exposure to a foreign substance (such as bee venom or drug reactivity). Emergency treatment includes epinephrine injections, used as a heart stimulant, vaso-constrictor, and bronchial relaxant.

Type II Hypersensitivity: Antibody-Mediated Hypersensitivity

Type II hypersensitivity reactions are due to antibodies directed against cell membrane–associated antigen. The end result of the antibody response is cytolysis. The mechanism may involve complement (*cytotoxic antibody*) or effector

lymphocytes that bind to target cell–associated antibody and effect cytolysis via a complement-independent pathway. In complement-mediated type II hypersensitivity, antibody recognition of cell-surface epitopes leads to assembly of the complement membrane attack complex (MAC, C5–C9) and

PHARMACOLOGY

Epinephrine

Epinephrine (adrenaline, $C_9H_{13}NO_3$) is a catecholamine hormone secreted by the adrenal medulla and released into the bloodstream in response to physical or mental stress. Epinephrine may be used to stimulate cardiac action in cardiac arrest, as a vasoconstrictor in anaphylactic shock, and as a bronchodilator in acute bronchial asthma. Chemically, epinephrine is a sympathomimetic monoamine derived from the amino acids phenylalanine and tyrosine.

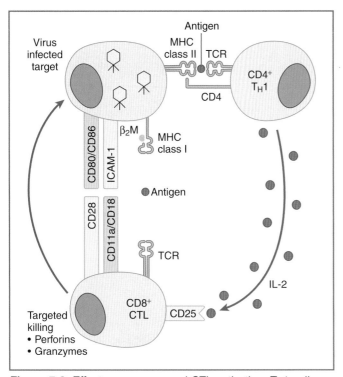

Figure 7-3. Effector response and CTL activation. T$_H$1 cells recognizing antigen presented through class II molecules drive CD8$^+$ cells to become activated cytotoxic cells (CTLs). Responses are mediated through IL-2 and the IL-2 receptor (CD25), and strengthened through interactions between the CTL and the infected target cell.

subsequent lysis of the cell. This reaction is the underlying mechanism in multiple disease states, including that seen in autoimmune hemolytic anemia, Goodpasture's syndrome (directed against basement membrane molecules), and Rh incompatibility leading to erythroblastosis fetalis. In rare cases, pharmaceutical agents, such as penicillin or chlorpromazine, can bind cells, forming a novel antigenic surface complex that provokes antibody production and type II cytotoxic reactions.

A second mechanism for Type II reactions is characterized by antibody-dependent cell-mediated cytotoxicity (ADCC) induced by natural killer (NK) cells recognizing IgG attached to target cells bearing antigen. The constant portion of the antibody (Fc region) is bound by Fc receptors on the NK cell, leading to perforin release and NK cell–mediated lysis (Fig. 7-5). Neutrophils, eosinophils, and macrophages may also participate in ADCC. ADCC may be involved in the pathophysiology of certain virus-induced immunologic diseases, such as those seen during active response to retroviral infection.

Type III Hypersensitivity: Immunocomplex-Mediated Hypersensitivity

Type III hypersensitivity results from soluble antigen-antibody immunocomplexes that activate complement (Fig. 7-6). The antigens may be self or foreign (i.e., microbial). Such complexes are deposited on membrane surfaces of various organs (e.g., kidney, lung, synovium). The byproducts of complement activation (C3a, C5a) are chemotaxins for

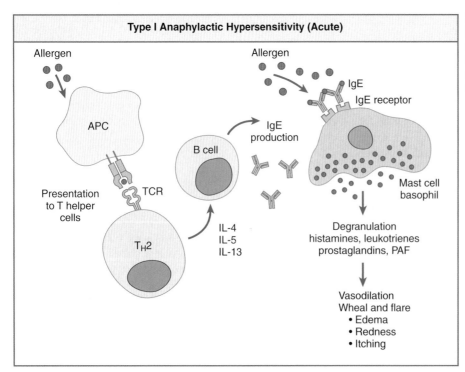

Figure 7-4. Type I acute anaphylactic hypersensitivity. Antibody-mediated cross-linking of allergens triggers mast cells or basophils to release vasoactive mediators, resulting in tissue damage and anaphylactic response.

Figure 7-5. Type II antibody-mediated hypersensitivity. Type II reactions can occur through antibody recognition of surface antigen and subsequent deposition of complement; lysis is mediated through assembly of the complement membrane attack complex (*left*). Alternatively, bound antibodies are cross-linked through Fc receptors on PMNs or NK cells, leading to antibody-dependent release of cytotoxic granules (*right*).

acute inflammatory cells, resulting in infiltration by polymorphonuclear cells. Lysosomal enzymes are released that result in tissue injury. Platelet aggregation occurs, resulting in microthrombus formation in the vasculature. This type of hypersensitivity was classically characterized as the *Arthus reaction*, identified by high degree of polymorphonuclear (PMN) infiltrate, vasoactive amine release, and erythema and edema in response to intradermal injection of antigen. Type III reactions and accompanying inflammatory injury are seen in diseases such as rheumatoid arthritis, systemic lupus erythematosus, and postinfectious arthritis.

Type IV Hypersensitivity: Delayed-Type (Cell-Mediated) Hypersensitivity

Type IV hypersensitivity (also called *delayed-type hypersensitivity*, DTH) involves T cell–antigen interactions that cause activation, cytokine secretion, and potential granuloma formation. This type of hypersensitivity requires sensitized lymphocytes that respond 24 to 48 hours after exposure to soluble antigen. DTH reactions may involve T_H cells (CD4+) or cytotoxic T cells (CD8+ CTLs). Diseases such as tuberculosis, leprosy, and sarcoidosis as well as contact dermatitis are all clinical examples where tissue injury is primarily due to the vigorous immune response to released antigens rather than to the inciting pathogen itself. In these examples, sustained release of antigen and continued activation of sensitized T cells result in amplified tissue damage. Continual antigen release due to persisting infection may provoke ex-

PATHOLOGY

Autoimmune Vasculitis

Autoimmune antibody-mediated diseases include rheumatoid arthritis, which exhibits chronic inflammation and vasculitis due to antibody-antigen complex deposition. The primary targets of inflammation are synovial membranes and articular structures; joint deformities and disability result from the erosion and destruction of synovial membranes and articular surfaces.

cessive macrophage activation and granulomatous responses, leading to extended fibrosis and necrosis of tissue.

A classic DTH reaction is exemplified in the tuberculin skin test (Mantoux reaction) (Fig. 7-7). An individual sensitized to tuberculosis through exposure or infection develops CD4+ lymphocytes specific for mycobacterial antigens. Skin testing through intradermal injection of purified protein derivative from mycobacteria (PPD) results in activation of sensitized CD4+ T cells. This is followed by secretion of cytokines, which cause recruitment and activation of macrophages. The result is localized reactivity manifested by erythema and induration within 48 hours.

In instances of viral infection, CD8+ cells react to antigens presented via class I MHC molecules. Cytotoxic cells recognize the presented antigen and lyse the infected target. Bystander killing may occur due to over-aggressive responses, such as those seen in smallpox, measles, and herpes infections.

Type III Immunocomplex-mediated Hypersensitivity

Figure 7-6. Type III immunocomplex-mediated hypersensitivity. Deposition of immunocomplexes in vascular beds results in platelet aggregation, complement fixation, and subsequent PMN infiltration. Released factors from activated PMNs cause significant tissue damage and pathology, mediated by formation of the complement cascade membrane attack complex (MAC) or via lysis by released cytotoxic granules.

Type IV Cell-mediated Hypersensitivity

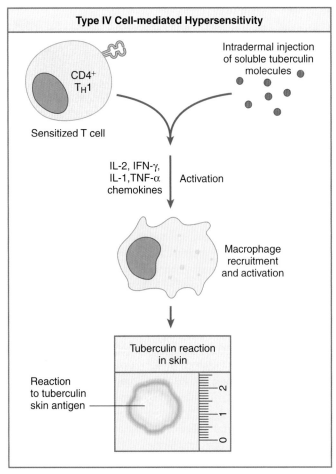

Figure 7-7. Type IV delayed-type (cell-mediated) hypersensitivity. The Mantoux tuberculin skin test is performed to evaluate whether a person has been exposed to tuberculosis. A positive reaction of more than 10 mm indicates reactivity of T cells with intradermal injected soluble mycobacterial antigen. This is manifested by induration and inflammation at the injection site.

KEY POINTS ABOUT HYPERSENSITIVITY

- Hypersensitivity reactions fall into four major categories:
- Type I reactions represent allergic reactions (anaphylactic hypersensitivity).
- Type II reactions are antibody mediated and are characterized by cytotoxic events.
- Type III reactions are characterized by immunocomplex deposition and subsequent tissue destruction.
- Type IV reactions represent delayed-type hypersensitive responses that are controlled in large part by T-cell reactivity to antigen.

Immunomodulation

8

CONTENTS

The regulation of immune function and overall immuno-homeostasis is under control of multiple factors that include genetic and environmental components. HLA allotypes, antigen dose, and existing cytokine milieu can all influence responses to pathogenic agents. Age, nutritional status, and status of neuroendocrine molecules can also contribute in a complex relationship to cellular response. At one extreme, newborns are immunocompetent but immune immature at birth; fetuses make IgM but not IgG until birth. Maternal IgG provides protection against bacterial agents through the first months of life. Extreme age also is a determinant. Immune senescence occurs in the elderly in whom good memory responses are available but poor primary (naïve) response results in increased susceptibility to organisms and strains never before encountered. Both nutritional status and stress-related endocrine changes directly affect cell-mediated immune responses, most often leading to immunosuppression.

●●● EVENTS INVOLVED IN T-LYMPHOCYTE ACTIVATION

Immune response must be regulated to be sufficient to protect the host without excessive or inappropriate responses (hypersensitivities) that may create disease. Activation of T cells requires two distinct signals: one through the TCR/CD3 complex when interacting with peptide on MHC and a second costimulatory signal. Receptor recognition of antigen mediates transcription of cytokine genes by a complex sequence of molecular events (Fig. 8-1). Absence of a second-ary signal can lead to cellular inactivation. The professional presenting cells that provide costimulation are dendritic cells, macrophages, and B cells. Of these cell types, dendritic cells deliver the best costimulatory signals for activation of naïve T cells. Presenting cells use the membrane molecules of the B7 family to deliver costimulatory signals through interaction with their ligand on T-cell membranes, CD28; two isoforms of the B7 family (B7.1 and B7.2; also called CD80 and CD86) act to regulate cytokine responses. For example, CD80 binding up-regulates T_H1 cytokines (IL-2, IFN-γ), while CD86 binding up-regulates T_H2 response (IL-4, IL-5, IL-6, and IL-10). Interactions with CD28 are critical in that binding to CD28 on the lymphocyte leads to IL-2 production, a major T-cell growth factor, whereas inhibition of binding leads to development of tolerance. Interaction of the B7 molecules with other T-cell surface antigens, such as CD152 (CTLA-4), leads to supressive signals and tolerance/anergy, or signaling induction of memory cell formation.

KEY POINTS ABOUT EVENTS INVOLVED IN T-LYMPHOCYTE ACTIVATION

- Immune responses are regulated to allow sufficient response without development of hypersensitivity.
- Activation of T cells requires two distinct signals: one by TCR recognition of MHC-presented antigen and another through costimulatory molecule interactions.

●●● TOLERANCE FOR SPECIFIC CONTROL OF IMMUNE RESPONSE

The major goal of the adaptive immune response is recognition of specific antigens, for which the specificity is controlled to allow recognition of foreign (non-self) antigens. The intensity and duration of response must be sufficient to protect against invading pathogens, with prompt and specific down-regulation when foreign antigen is no longer present. "Immunologic tolerance" is the failure to mount an immune

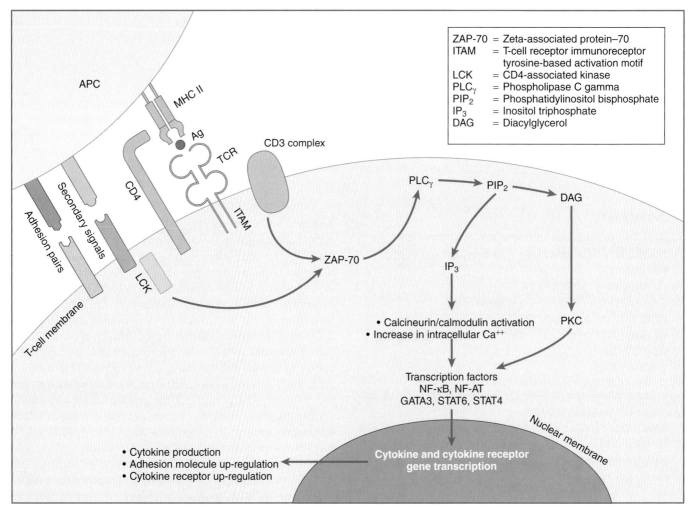

Figure 8-1. Receptor-mediated transcription of cytokine genes by a sequence of molecular events. T-cell receptors recognizing antigen presented by MHC molecules triggers transduction of signals across the cell membrane through the CD3 complex, resulting in up-regulation of T-cell activation genes (cytokines and cytokine receptors).

response to an antigen. Immunologic tolerance is not simply the failure to recognize an antigen but rather an active response to a particular epitope that allows specific unresponsiveness while the rest of the host response remains intact and capable of response.

Tolerance of Lymphocytes

Tolerance can be at the level of B or T lymphocytes, or both, and can be accomplished by a variety of mechanisms including apoptosis, anergy, antigen excess, and suppressor T-cell formation (Fig. 8-2). T-regulatory cells also play a role in modification of immune development and response. Only lymphocytes bearing antigen receptors can be tolerized. Tolerance can be induced early during adaptive cell development, or peripherally during maturation of response. Two mechanisms for tolerance include *apoptosis*, or programmed cell deletion, and *anergy*, a state of clonal inactivation due to lack of secondary signals.

Elimination of Self-Reactive Lymphocytes

Induction of tolerance in immature lymphocytes is critical for elimination of self-reactive cells. For T lymphocytes, negative selection via apoptosis in the thymus eliminates the majority of cells that bear high reactivity to self-peptides. Mature cells leaving the thymus may also be tolerized, subject to antigenic factors that affect immunogenicity. Factors that induce tolerance include extremely high- or low-dose antigen, weak MHC binding, and route of administration (e.g., oral antigens are well tolerated). Peripheral tolerance occurs primarily via anergic reactions, where costimulatory signals provided by B7 on the surface of the presenting cell are absent. Finally, tolerance may also occur in immunologically privileged sites, such as the eye, brain, and testes, usually due to local secretion of immunosuppressive factors (e.g., TGF-β) that down-regulate response. The developing fetus in the uterus is a prime example of a privileged site in which recognition to foreign antigen is suppressed.

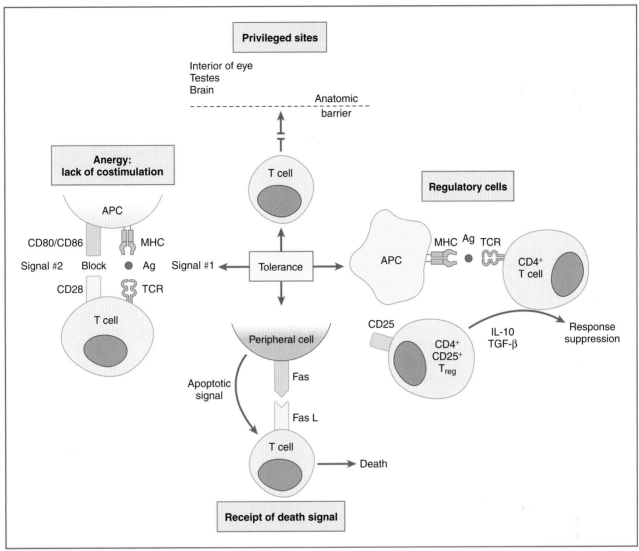

Figure 8-2. Mechanisms of tolerance. Tolerance can occur by mechanisms including apoptosis of reactive cells, development of anergic response to antigen through loss of secondary signals, regulation of response as a result of antigen excess, and active suppression by regulatory T cells.

ANATOMY & EMBRYOLOGY

Apoptosis Vascular Development

The development of vasculature to serve as a nutrient and waste pipeline is fundamental for organ development embryogenesis. Although the molecular determinants of capillary regression are as yet unresolved, apoptosis as a mechanism for cell death is critical in fetal development for regionalization of mesoderm in embryonic growth.

Immature B cells in the bone marrow undergo apoptosis upon recognition of self-antigens by activation-induced cell death mechanisms. Alternatively, the B cell may undergo receptor editing to change the binding specificity of the surface immunoglobulin, thus rendering the cell no longer self-reactive. Once in the peripheral tissue, B cells may undergo an anergic response dependent upon the level of specific antigen. Low-dose soluble monomeric antigens do not permit receptor cross-linking on the surface of the B cell, sending signals to clonally inactivate the B cell. An excessively high antigen dose also can result in anergic response owing to overwhelming recognition in the absence of sufficient T-cell costimulation. Finally, self-reactive B cells that escape elimination or induction of anergy may be incapable of activation as a result of the lack of T cells available to help initiate development of autoimmune response.

KEY POINTS ABOUT TOLERANCE FOR SPECIFIC CONTROL OF IMMUNE RESPONSE

- Immunologic tolerance represents specific unresponsiveness to antigen while remaining responses are intact.
- Factors influencing the nature, intensity, and duration of immune function include age, neuroendocrine hormone levels, HLA allotypes, antigen dose, and cytokine milieu.

■ Tolerance can be at the level of B or T lymphocytes, or both, and can be accomplished by mechanisms including apoptosis, anergy, antigen excess, and suppressor/regulatory T-cell formation.

●●● ETIOLOGY OF AUTOIMMUNE DISEASE

Failure of tolerance can lead to development of autoimmunity. It is clear that environmental and genetic components are risk factors for disease. Genetic factors have been identified (polymorphisms of cytokine genes, such as TNF, or their receptors; apoptosis genes; complement component deficiencies), and others are likely to be revealed soon. In addition, infections or exogenous agents that cause physical damage are likely to also play important roles. The mechanisms underlying all autoimmune diseases are not fully elucidated; however, genetic polymorphisms of MHC class II genes (alleles of HLA-DR and/or HLA-DQ) are associated with increased susceptibility to autoimmune diseases. Possible mechanisms for a loss of tolerance leading to autoimmune reactions include (1) a lack of Fas-Fas ligand–mediated deletion of autoreactive T cells in the thymus during development, (2) loss of T-regulatory or T-cell suppressor function, (3) cross-reactivity between exogenous and self-antigens (molecular mimicry), (4) excessive B-cell function due to polyclonal activation by exogenous factors (of viral or bacterial origin), (5) abnormal expression of MHC class II molecules by cells that normally do not express these surface molecules, and (6) release of sequestered self-antigens from privileged sites, thus priming for responses not previously seen by the immune system.

Autoimmune diseases can be classified as organ specific or systemic in nature (Table 8-1). Three major types of autoimmune reaction mechanisms are recognized as causing different autoimmune disorders (Fig. 8-3). Two of these mechanisms involve autoantibodies directed against self-antigens; for both, classical complement pathway activation exacerbates local damage and inflammatory response. In the first case, autoantibodies may be directed against a specific

PATHOLOGY & NEUROSCIENCE

Multiple Sclerosis

Multiple sclerosis is a demyelinating disease of the central nervous system, leading to patches of sclerosis (plaques) in the brain and spinal cord. The pathology is caused by T-cell responses directed against antigens of the myelin basic protein. Early clinical manifestations are dependent upon the location and size of the plaque, with common symptoms including visual loss and diplopia, slurred speech (dysarthria), muscle weakness, and abnormal touch sensation (paresthesia).

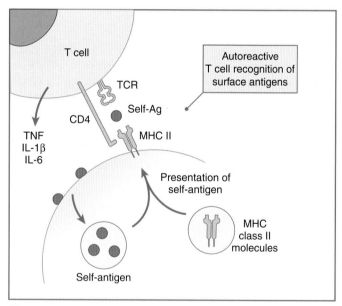

Figure 8-3. Autoimmunity and disease.

self-component, such as a surface molecule or receptor. Examples include antibodies against the acetylcholine receptor producing myasthenia gravis, and antithyroid-stimulating hormone receptor antibodies producing Graves' disease. Autoantibodies may also bind with antigens present in the blood, forming antigen-antibody (immune) complexes that later deposit in organs, thus inciting an inflammatory response. An example is seen in lupus glomerulonephritis in which complexes of anti-DNA antibodies and free DNA accumulate in the kidney. The third mechanism is that of

TABLE 8-1. Autoimmunity and Disease

Autoimmune Disease	Mechanism	Pathology
Autoimmune hemolytic anemia	Autoantibodies to RBC antigens	Lysis of RBCs and anemia
Autoimmune thrombocytopenia purpura	Autoantibodies to platelet integrin	Bleeding, abnormal platelet function
Myasthenia gravis	Autoantibodies to acetylcholine receptor in neuromuscular junction	Blockage of neuromuscular junction transmission and muscle weakness
Graves' disease	Autoantibodies to receptor for thyroid-stimulating hormone (TSH)	Stimulation of increased release of thyroid hormone (hyperthyroidism)
Hashimoto's thyroiditis	Autoantibodies and autoreactive T cells to thyroglobulin and thyroid microsomal antigens	Destruction of thyroid gland (hypothyroidism)
Type I diabetes (insulin-dependent diabetes mellitus; IDDM)	Autoantibodies and autoreactive T cells to pancreatic islet cells	Destruction of islet cells and failure of insulin production
Goodpasture's syndrome	Autoantibodies to type IV collagen	Glomerulonephritis
Rheumatic fever	Autoantibodies to cardiac myosin (cross-reactive to streptococcal cell wall component)	Myocarditis
Pemphigus vulgaris	Autoantibodies to epidermal components (cadherin, desmoglein)	Acantholytic dermatosis, skin blistering
Multiple sclerosis	T-cell response against myelin basic protein	Demyelination, marked by patches of hardened tissue in the brain or the spinal cord; partial or complete paralysis and jerking muscle tremor
Systemic lupus erythematosus (SLE)	Circulating immunocomplexes deposited in skin, kidneys, etc, formed by autoantibodies to nuclear antigens (antinuclear antibodies, or ANA), including anti-DNA	Glomerulitis, arthritis, vasculitis, skin rash
Rheumatoid arthritis	Autoantibodies to IgG (rheumatoid factors); deposition of immunocomplexes in synovium of joints and elsewhere; infiltrating autoreactive T cells in synovium	Joint inflammation, destruction of cartilage and bone

autoreactive T cells that recognize targeted self-antigens on organs, leading to direct damage to tissue. In many cases, autoreactive T cells coexist with autoantibody responses, leading to exacerbation of disease and organ damage. In the case of multiple sclerosis, T cells reactive to myelin basic protein destroy the protective layer surrounding axons, thereby eliminating effective transfer of signals through nerves.

KEY POINTS ABOUT THE ETIOLOGY OF AUTOIMMUNE DISEASE

- Autoimmunity represents a failure of effective tolerance to self-antigens.
- Genetic and environmental factors play a role in the etiology of disease.
- Mechanisms of disease include autoantibodies that are directed against specific self-components, deposition of circulating antibody-antigen complexes, and deleterious responses by autoreactive T cells.

●●● TRANSPLANTATION: CONTROL OF IMMUNE-MEDIATED REJECTION

Graft Tissue

Understanding of the mechanisms involved in immuno-regulation has allowed increased success rates of tissue transplantation in the clinic. It has long been known that tissue transplanted from an individual to another location within the same individual (*autografts*) is well tolerated. Similarly, organs transplanted between identical twins or animals from an inbred strain of the same species (*syngeneic grafts* or *isografts*) have a high degree of success. By contrast, grafts transplanted between individuals of different species (*xenografts* or *heterografts*) are rarely successful without a high degree of immunosuppression. Indeed, grafts made between genetically different individuals of the same species (*allografts* or *homografts*) are tolerated only when major histocompatibility antigens are matched. The common cause of graft rejection is due to Tcell recognition of foreign HLA antigens on the donor tissue. Histocompatibility testing is used to identify HLA class I and class II antigens, as a measure to maximize the number of alleles conserved between donor and recipient individuals. Alloreactivity may therefore be defined as the stimulation of host T-cell responses against foreign HLA antigens. However, even with a high degree of HLA similarity, minor (non-HLA) alloantigens may induce rejection of allografts.

Mechanisms of Allograft Rejection

The mechanisms for allograft rejection are defined by the speed at which the tissue is attacked by the host (Fig. 8-4). Hyperacute rejection occurs within minutes after tissue transplantation and is mediated by preformed antibodies present and directed against HLA or blood group antigens. Antibodies bound to vasculature activate complement components, causing immediate obstruction and destruction of donor blood vessels. This is in contrast to acute rejection, in which T cells responding to donor tissue antigens are amplified and activated. Acute rejection occurs approximately 10 to 30 days after tissue implantation. Even if tissue is matched for major histocompatibility antigens, the minor HLA components may be enough to eventually cause rejection of tissue. Chronic rejection, therefore, manifests as reactions occurring months to years after transplantation, involving both T cells and antibodies directed against minor antigens; infiltration of CD4+ and CD8+ T cells causes release of cytokines and direct lysis of target tissue, eventually resulting in graft rejection.

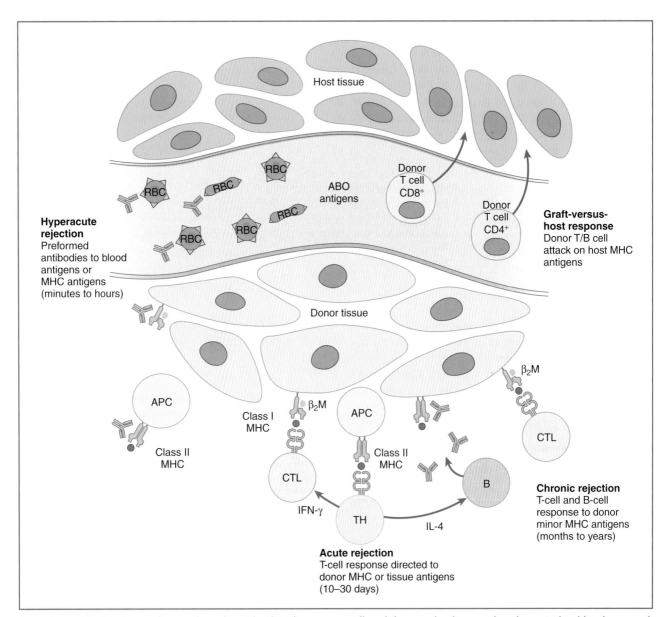

Figure 8-4. Mechanisms of transplantation rejection. Immune-mediated tissue rejection can be characterized by the speed of response to donor tissue and the effector mechanisms involved.

TABLE 8-2. Immunosuppressive Agents Used in Clinical Transplantation

Immunosuppressive Agent	Structure	Mechanism of Action
Cyclosporine (CsA)	Cyclic polypeptide produced by *Tolypocladium inflatum*	Inhibits T_H lymphocytes; blocks production of IL-2, IFN-γ, and IL-4; binds to cytoplasmic immunophilin to inhibit calcineurin, affecting nuclear factors and preventing cytokine gene transcription
Tacrolimus (TCL; FK506)	Macrolide produced by *Streptomyces tsukubaensis*	Forms a complex with FK-binding protein; also blocks calcineurin function and prevents IL-2 (and other cytokine) gene transcription
Sirolimus (SRL)	Macrolide antibiotic produced by *Streptomyces hygroscopicus*	Inhibits cytokine signal transduction (e.g., IL-2 receptor signaling)
Azathioprine (AZA)	S-imidazole derivative of 6-mercaptopurine	Inhibits de novo DNA synthesis, affecting initiation of primary immune responses
Corticosteroids	Synthetic glucocorticoids and analogs	Depresses T-lymphocyte activity
Polyclonal antilymphocyte serum	Prepared in animals directed against human lymphocytes	Lowers numbers of circulating lymphocytes

Immunosuppressive Agents to Prevent Allograft Rejection

At present there is no clinical protocol to induce complete tolerance to allografts. Therefore, all patients require daily treatment with immunosuppressive agents. All immunosuppressive agents in clinical use have drawbacks relating either to toxicity and side effects or to failure to provide sufficient immunosuppression. On the one hand, excessive immunosuppression can lead to development of opportunistic infections and neoplasia. On the other hand, inadequate immunosuppression allows the recipient to mount an immune response, causing allograft rejection. Table 8-2 lists immunosuppressive agents used in clinical transplantation.

Graft-Versus-Host Disease

One consequence of increased graft acceptance due to immunosuppressive drugs is graft-versus-host disease (GVHD). A "reverse rejection" occurs whereby healthy donor lymphocytes recognize the patient's tissues as foreign. In GVHD, persistent lymphocytes proliferate and react against the host antigens; over time, this expanded population targets the skin, bowel, and liver, as well as other tissues.

PATHOLOGY

Graft-Versus-Host Disease

T cells expanded from within an allogeneic donor organ transplant (e.g., bone marrow transplant) react against the recipient's antigens, attacking cells and tissues. Disease extends to affect the skin, gastrointestinal tract, and liver, with symptoms including rash, fever, diarrhea, liver dysfunction, abdominal pain, and anorexia.

●●● IMMUNODEFICIENCY DISORDERS AS A PREDISPOSITION TO INFECTION

Immunodeficiency disorders are a diverse group of illnesses that result from one or more abnormalities of the immune system (Fig. 8-5). The abnormalities can involve absence or malfunction of blood cells (lymphocytes, granulocytes, monocytes) or soluble molecules (antibodies, complement components) and can result from an inherited genetic trait (primary) or from an unrelated illness or treatment (secondary). The principal manifestation of immunodeficiency is an increased susceptibility to infection as documented by increased frequency or severity of infection, prolonged duration of infection with development of an unexpected complication or unusual manifestation, or infection with organisms of low pathogenicity.

KEY POINTS ABOUT IMMUNODEFICIENCY DISORDERS AS A PREDISPOSITION TO INFECTION

- Immunodeficiencies lead to disease susceptibility dependent upon loss of immune function.
- B-cell deficiency is marked by recurrent infections with encapsulated bacteria.
- T-cell deficiency manifests as recurrent viral, fungal, or protozoal infections.
- Phagocytic deficiency with the associated inability to engulf and destroy pathogens usually appears with recurrent bacterial infections.
- Complement disorders demonstrate defects in activation patterns of the classical, alternative, and/or lectin-binding pathways, which augment adaptive host defense mechanisms.

Immunodeficiency			
B-Cell Deficiencies		**T-Cell Deficiencies**	
Recurrent bacterial infections		*Severe viral, fungal, and protozoal infections*	
Bruton's agammaglobulinemia—defect in B-cell development	**B and T-cell deficiencies**	Bare lymphocyte syndrome—lack of class II MHC	
Common variable–hypogammaglobulinemia—defect in plasma cell differentiation	Severe combined immunodeficiency	Omenn's syndrome—defect in TCR gene rearrangement	
Hyper-IgM syndrome—defect in class switching		DiGeorge syndrome—thymic aplasia	
Phagocytic Cell Deficiencies		**Complement Deficiencies**	
Recurrent bacterial infections		*Recurrent bacterial infections* *Defects in immunocomplex clearance*	
Chronic granulomatous disease—lack of respiratory burst		C1, C2, or C4 deficiency—defects in clearing immunocomplexes	
Leukocyte adhesion deficiency—lack of PMN extravasation into tissue		C3 or C5 deficiency—block in alternative and classical pathways	
Chediak-Higashi syndrome—defect in neutrophil microtubule function and related phagosome/lysosome fusion		C6, C7, C8, or C9—defect in MAC assembly and function	

Figure 8-5. Primary immunodeficiencies. Manifestation of immunodeficiency is dependent upon the etiology of response. B-cell deficiency is marked by recurrent infections with encapsulated bacteria. T-cell deficiency manifests as recurrent viral, fungal, or protozoal infections. Phagocytic deficiency with associated inability to engulf and destroy pathogens usually appears with recurrent bacterial infections. Complement disorders demonstrate defects in activation patterns of the classical, alternative, and/or lectin-binding pathways, which augment adaptive host defense mechanisms.

●●● IMMUNOPROPHYLAXIS AGAINST INFECTIOUS AGENTS

The active process of exposure to infectious agents or their antigenic components (vaccination or immunoprophylaxis) has been one of the most important medical advances that directly affect longevity and quality of life. Immunization may be characterized as active, whereby exposure to antigen generates protective immunity of the host, or as passive, in which administered humoral (antibody) or cellular factors confer host resistance to disease. Active immunization provides long-lasting immunity, whereas passive administration of factors leads to fast-acting but temporary immunity to eminent or ongoing exposure.

Vaccination schedules require understanding of the immune status of the developing individual (Table 8-3). The fetus begins to produce IgM at 6 months' gestation; most IgG at birth is transplacental and maternal in origin. Infants do not respond well to polysaccharide antigens prior to 2 years of age (Fig. 8-6). Antigenicity of small molecules (haptens) improves when they are conjugated to protein. Vaccines also contain *adjuvants*, which are excipients included in the vaccine formulation to stimulate immune function toward production of protective responses against pathogenic antigens.

TABLE 8-3. Schedule for Active Immunization of Children and Adults

Age	Vaccine
Birth	Hepatitis B (Hep B)
1–2 months	Hep B
2 months	Diphtheria and tetanus toxoids and acellular pertussis (DTP), *Haemophilus influenzae* type b (Hib), inactivated poliovirus (IPV)
4 months	DTP, Hib, IPV, rotavirus (Rv)
6 months	Hep B, DTP, Hib, IPV, Rv
12–15 months	Oral poliovirus vaccine (OPV); measles, mumps, rubella (MMR); varicella vaccine for susceptible children
4–6 years	DTP, OPV, MMR
11–12 years	Hep B, MMR, varicella
25–64 years	Measles, rubella
>65 years	Influenza, pneumococcal disease

KEY POINTS ABOUT IMMUNOPROPHYLAXIS AGAINST INFECTIOUS AGENTS

- Immunization may be active or passive.
- Active immunity is the development of antibodies in response to antigenic stimulation.
- Passive immunity is transferred protection through preformed antibodies produced by another individual.

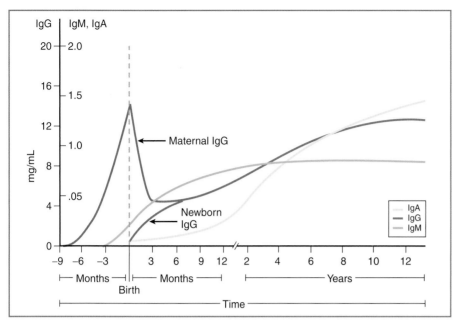

Figure 8-6. Developmental progression of antibody isotypes. Maternal antibodies wane through the first year as the child produces antibodies of his or her own.

Immunoassays

9

CONTENTS

Immunoassays and experimental systems are designed to assist in the assessment of pathogenic responses and are instrumental in our understanding of the pathophysiology of diseases. The exquisite specificity of the antibody allows its use as an efficient analytical tool in biomedical research and diagnostic investigation. Cellular assays allow determination of lymphocyte function, and gene expression arrays allow in silica identification of molecular mechanisms that form the basis of disease.

●●● INTERACTIONS BETWEEN POLYCLONAL ANTIBODIES AND MULTIVALENT ANTIGENS

The use of antibodies has expanded from simple diagnostics to elucidation of gene function, localization of gene products, and rapid screening of biological effectors for drug discovery and testing. The interactions between antigen and antibody form the basis of many quantitative and qualitative diagnostic assays that involve noncovalent binding of antigenic determinants (*epitopes*) to the variable regions of both the heavy and the light immunoglobulin chains. These interactions are analogous to those observed in enzyme-substrate interactions and can be defined similarly through physical laws of mass action. Specifically, the reversible interaction between antibody and an antigen can be represented by the equation:

$$K = \frac{k_1}{k_{-1}} = \frac{[AbAg]}{[Ab][Ag]}$$

where K represents the equilibrium constant, k_1 is the association constant, k_{-1} is the dissociation constant, [Ab] represents the free antibody concentration, [Ag] represents the free antigen concentration, and [AbAg] represents complexed antibody with antigen.

Although each individual antibody is highly specific for antigenic structures, the population of serum antibodies is typically polyclonal in nature. This means that complex antigens give rise to multiple antibodies that react with different determinants inherent within the antigen. Because serum (IgG) antibodies are bivalent in their reactions with antigen, and because antigens are often multivalent in their interactions with antibodies, there exists a natural capacity for polyclonal antibodies to cross-link antigens.

●●● ANTIBODY-ANTIGEN INTERACTIONS: THE BASIS OF QUANTITATIVE AND QUALITATIVE ASSAYS

Experimentally, if a known concentration of antibody is mixed with increasing amounts of specific antigen, cross-

---

BIOCHEMISTRY

Affinity Constants

Affinity constants determining antibody-antigen interactions may be determined by analysis of the equilibrium association or dissociation constants. The equilibrium association constant and valence of an antibody can be found using the Scatchard equation, $r/c = K(n - r)$, where r is the moles of bound ligand per mole of antibody at equilibrium; c is the free ligand concentration at equilibrium; K is the equilibrium association constant; and n is the number of antigen-binding sites per antibody molecule.

linked antibody-antigen complexes begin to precipitate from the solution. Because of the nature of the number of potential binding sites, an equivalence zone of maximal precipitation can be determined that is characteristic of the interaction. If greater amounts of antigen are further added, the complexes will begin to dissolve and return to solution (Fig. 9-1). As discussed in Chapter 3, the antigen-antibody reactions are defined by *noncovalent forces*, *affinity*, and *avidity*.

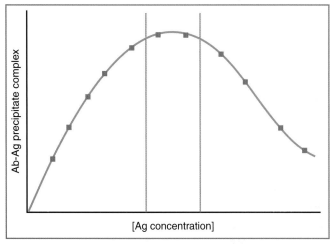

Figure 9-1. Physical interactions dictate antibody-antigen interactions.

The antibody titer reflects the measured amount of antibodies (in the blood), described as a relative dilution factor against a particular type of antigen (tissue, cell, or substance). Antibodies directed against epitopes on multideterminant antigens lead to agglutination reactions. The most widely known agglutination reaction is the *Coombs' test*, originally used to detect autoantibodies against host red blood cells (RBCs) (Fig. 9-2). Many diseases and drugs (e.g., quinidine, methyldopa, and procainamide) can lead to production of these antibodies, with repercussions of RBC destruction and resultant anemia. In direct agglutination tests, the agglutinating antibodies directly react with antigens on the surface of bacterial cells (*Brucella* and tularemia febrile agglutinin tests) or erythrocytes (direct hemagglutination test) to form visible clumps of particles. In passive hemagglutination tests, agglutinating antibodies react with antigens coupled to carrier particles such as erythrocytes (indirect or passive hemagglutination test) or gelatinous beads to form visible aggregates.

⬤⬤⬤ ANTIBODY-ANTIGEN PRECIPITATION REACTIONS IN GELS

Often, precipitation reactions are used for analysis in situations in which only qualitative detection is required. Reactions can be performed in a gel matrix to limit the rate of diffusion of reactants and hold the precipitate so that it is effectively immobilized for visualization. Several methods are widely used in medicine for analysis of hormones, enzymes, toxins, and immune system products.

Double Diffusion Assay (Ouchterlony Assay)

The double diffusion assay, also known as the Ouchterlony assay, was developed in the 1950s and is still in widespread use. The method is extremely simple and allows determination of identity (relatedness) between reagents. The most widespread use of the Ouchterlony technique is for comparison of antigens (Fig. 9-3). It is used in forensic medicine and in a variety of diagnostic assays.

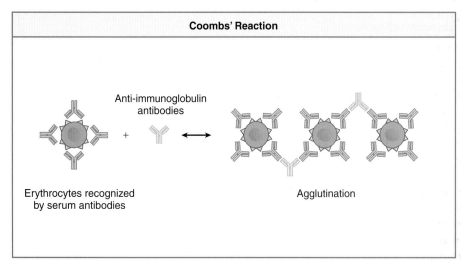

Coombs' Reaction

Anti-immunoglobulin antibodies

Erythrocytes recognized by serum antibodies

Agglutination

Figure 9-2. Coombs' reaction. Antibody recognition can be used to agglutinate large antigens, either directly or indirectly through cross-linking with anti-immunoglobulin antibodies. Pictured is an indirect Coombs' reaction in which autoantibodies recognizing determinants on erythrocytes are agglutinated using reactive anti-immunoglobulin antibodies.

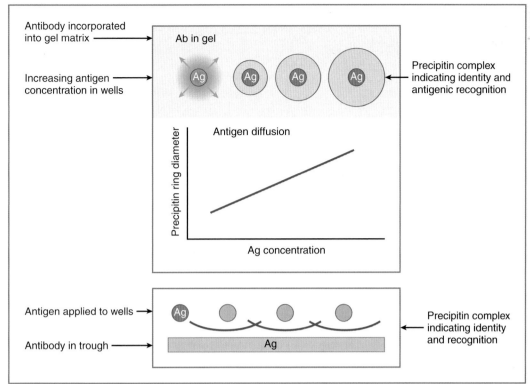

Figure 9-3. Double diffusion assay. The Ouchterlony assay (*top*) is characterized by precipitin reactions occurring as applied antigen diffuses through a gel matrix containing reactive antibodies. The diameter of the precipitin ring formed can be quantitated by comparison to known standard antigen concentrations. The radial diffusion assay (*bottom*) allows qualitative determination as antibody and antigen diffuse toward each other through the assay matrix.

Radial Immunodiffusion Assay

A variation of the double diffusion assay allows quantitative measurement of antigen. The radial immunodiffusion assay (see Fig. 9-3) incorporates antibody directly into the assay gel matrix. Antigen is applied to wells and allowed to diffuse through the gel. A precipitin ring forms as the antigen and antibody interact; the amount of antigen applied to the well is proportional to the diameter of the precipitin ring. Comparison of unknown samples to known antigen concentrations allows quantitative analysis.

●●● MONOCLONAL AND POLYCLONAL ANTIBODY SPECIFICITY FOR ANTIGEN DETECTION

Antibodies in serum are by nature polyclonal, with potential to recognize more than 10^{14} different antigenic epitopes. Exposure to foreign molecules (non-self), either by infection or by immunization, will increase the relative balance and titer of polyclonal antibodies toward a specific antigen. Monoclonal antibodies are well suited as diagnostic reagents for sensitive and specific detection of defined molecular epitopes.

Western Blot (Immunoblotting) Detection of Membrane-Bound Antigens

A mixture of proteins (e.g., antigens derived from pathogenic organisms) may be separated by electrophoresis through a gel matrix and then transferred onto a solid medium such as nitrocellulose that binds proteins tightly. Antibodies with a reporter enzyme covalently attached are incubated with proteins bound to the nitrocellulose. Substrate for the enzyme is added, which turns colors when enzyme is present. The resulting colored line demonstrates that the antigen was present in the initial population of mixed proteins. This type of test is clinically useful for detection of patient antibodies reactive to viral antigens, such as the *gag*, *pol*, or *env* gene products produced by the human immunodeficiency virus (HIV) (Fig. 9-4).

Enzyme-Linked Immunosorbent Assay (ELISA)

The two general approaches to diagnosing disease by immunoassay include methods that directly test for specific antigens or indirectly test for the presence of antigens by looking for antigen-specific antibodies. Enzyme-linked immunosorbent assays (ELISAs), also known as enzyme immunoassays (EIAs) or solid-phase immunoassays, are designed to detect antigens or antibodies by producing an enzyme-triggered color change. ELISAs are referred to as solid-phase assays because they require the immobilization of antigens or antibodies on solid surfaces. The noncompetitive ELISA utilizes a specific antigen attached to a solid-phase surface (plastic bead or microtiter well) (Fig. 9-5). The test specimen is added; incubation allows antibodies in the test specimen to bind to the antigen. A secondary enzyme-labeled antibody is used to detect the test antibody. A chromogenic substrate is added; the enzyme converts the substrate to a detectable colored compound. The amount of color that

Figure 9-4. Western blot (immunoblotting). Reactivity to antigens can be assessed by Western blot analysis. An example of detection using serum antibodies is pictured. HIV antigens separated by gel electrophoresis are transferred to a solid matrix (nitrocellulose), then probed with patient serum. Reactive antibodies against HIV antigens are visualized, thus determining patient exposure to the viral agent.

develops is proportional to the amount of antibody in the test specimen.

A similar assay employs an antigen-specific antibody bound to the well. The test specimen is added, and any specific antigen is captured by the immobilized antibody. A second enzyme-linked antibody, which binds a different antigenic determinant on the antigen, is then added to detect captured antigen. In this format, the antigen is "sandwiched" between antibodies. Similarly to the noncompetitive ELISA, the amount of color produced in the presence of enzyme-labeled reporter is proportional to the antigen in the test specimen.

Immunohistochemical Methods

Antibody-based assays can be used to determine whether a particular antigen is found on or in the cells of a particular tissue. The method involves covalent attachment of reporter enzymes or fluorescent tags to specific antibodies to detect antigens. The enzyme horseradish peroxidase is frequently used as a coupled reagent, allowing deposition of diamino-benzidine for visualization of target cells (Fig. 9-6). Similarly, fluorochrome-tagged antibodies (fluorescein-, pycoerythrin-, rhodamine-, or allophycocyanin-conjugated antibodies) can be used to visualize antigen location after excitation with ultraviolet light.

Alternatively, a two-step method may be used in which unlabeled antibody specific for the antigen in question is reacted first with the tissue, followed by a tagged secondary antibody that recognizes the first specific antibody. Under these circumstances, the initial signal can be amplified, since multiple signals are generated by secondary antibodies that bind the primary antibody. The use of these antibodies with fluorescent tags, in concert with advances in microscopy, has transformed disease research. For example, immunofluo-rescence is widely used in clinical laboratories for screening patients' sera for anti-DNA antibodies in suspected cases of systemic lupus erythematosus.

Fluorescence-Activated Cell Sorting (FACS)

FACS analysis is used to identify, and sometimes purify, one cell subset from a mixture of cells (Fig. 9-7). Antibodies directed against surface molecules can be used to identify and quantitatively analyze specific cell phenotypes within a population of cells. Antibodies may be directly tagged with fluorescent molecules or indirectly identified with secondary tagging (indirect immunofluorescence). Labeled cells are passed single-file through a laser beam by continuous flow in a fine suspension stream. Each cell scatters some of the laser light. Detection of scattered light in a parallel manner (forward scatter) is indicative of cell size, whereas detection of scattered light at a perpendicular angle (side scatter) is indicative of cellular granularity. These physical parameters alone can distinctly identify granular PMNs, mononuclear cells, and RBCs. Antibody-labeled cells emit fluorescent light when excited by the laser. Cells are detected at an extremely rapid rate of data acquisition. Newer methodologies allow detection of intracellular cytokines to match cytokine production within individual cell phenotypes.

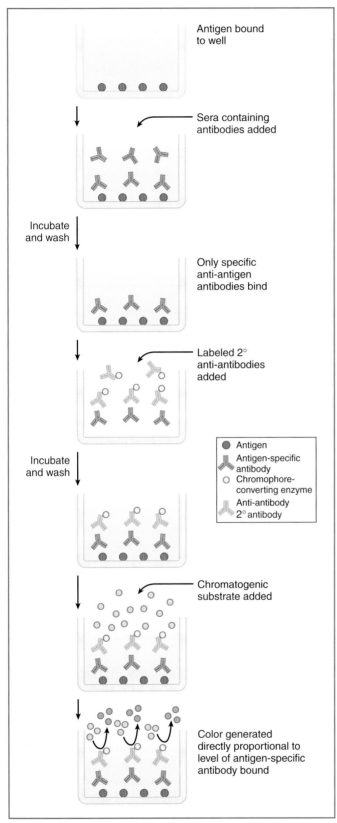

Antigen bound
to well

Sera containing
antibodies added

Incubate
and wash

Only specific
anti-antigen
antibodies bind

Labeled 2°
anti-antibodies
added

Incubate
and wash

Chromatogenic
substrate added

Color generated
directly proportional to
level of antigen-specific
antibody bound

● Antigen
Y Antigen-specific
antibody
○ Chromophore-
converting enzyme
Y Anti-antibody
2° antibody

Figure 9-5. Enzyme-linked immunosorbent assay (ELISA). Serum added to wells coated with antigen is probed with antibodies. Enzyme-conjugated secondary antibodies detect the primary complex. Catalytic conversion of chromogenic substrate allows quantitation against known standards.

Figure 9-6. Immunohistochemical method. Use of antibodies to identify cell structure and phenotype within tissue is a powerful tool. Pictured are lymphocytes cuffing pulmonary vascular regions. Arrows indicate localized CD3$^+$ lymphocytes in tissue. Enzyme (horseradish peroxidase)–conjugated antibodies directed against surface CD3$^+$ were incubated with the tissue section. Conversion and subsequent deposition of chromogenic substrate (diaminobenzidine) enable identification and visualization of T lymphocytes.

●●● ASSAYS TO DETERMINE IMMUNE FUNCTION

Complement Fixation Test

The complement fixation test is a blood test in which a sample of serum is exposed to a particular antigen and complement to determine whether antibodies to that particular antigen are present (Fig. 9-8). The nature of complement is to react in combination with antigen-antibody complexes. The relative lack of antigen specificity allows complement to react with almost any antigen-antibody complex. In the test procedure, complement remains free unless fixed by the particular antigen and antibody system in question. The indicator used in many complement fixation assays is sheep RBCs. In a positive or reactive test, the complement is bound to an antigen-antibody complex and is not free to interact with target RBCs. The RBCs remain unlysed and settle to the bottom of a concave-shaped well to form a button. In a negative or nonreactive test, the complement remains free to interact with the blood cells, causing them to lyse. The complement test is a powerful tool to identify antibodies reacting with antigens to confirm exposure to a specific microorganism. For example, the Wasserman reaction is an example of a diagnostic complement fixation test to detect antibodies to the syphilis organism *Treponema pallidum*; a positive reaction indicates the presence of antibodies and therefore syphilis infection.

Figure 9-7. Fluorescence-activated cell sorting. Flow cytometric analysis allows direct identification of cell phenotypes using fluorescently tagged antibody molecules. Modern cytometers can measure multiple parameters simultaneously, including low-angle forward scatter (proportional to cell diameter), orthogonal scatter intensity (measuring cellular granularity), as well as fluorescence intensity at several wavelengths (**A**). Pictured is a scattergram of splenocytes screened for reactivity with an FITC-labeled anti-CD3 antibody to allow quantitation of T lymphocytes within the population (**B**). A shift to the right on the x-axis indicates the presence of positively stained cells with increasing CD3 surface molecule present. FITC, fluorescein isothiocyanate; SSC, side scatter.

Lymphocyte Function Assays

Lymphocyte function assays can determine the state of B- or T-cell responsiveness to specific or nonspecific antigens. Investigation of mitogenic activation is a useful diagnostic tool to establish basic cellular function. Activation is accurately measured by way of blast transformation assay as a measure of in vitro reactivity (Fig. 9-9). Lipopolysaccharides (LPS) cause polyclonal stimulation of B cells in vitro. Several lectins, including concanavalin A (ConA) and phytohemagglutinin (PHA) are effective T-cell mitogens. Pokeweed mitogen stimulates polyclonal activation of both B and T cells. For each cell type, a linear relationship between cell number and incorporated analog is established, enabling accurate, straightforward quantification of changes in proliferation.

Additional lymphocyte function assays include the mixed leukocyte reaction (MLR), in which inactivated recipient cells are mixed with donor lymphocytes to indicate whether CD4$^+$ cells of a recipient individual react to class II MHC of the donor. These assays are extremely powerful tools to assist in determination of transplant compatibility. Cytotoxicity assays measure the ability of cytotoxic T cells or NK cells to kill labeled target cells that express a specific antigen for which the cytotoxic T cells may be sensitive.

Microarrays to Assess Gene Expression

Levels of expression of thousands of genes can be measured simultaneously using a technology called *gene chips* or *microarrays*. Briefly, thousands of short complementary DNA (cDNA) samples representing genes from all parts of the genome are attached to a slide. Samples of messenger RNA (mRNA) from cells in culture are used and reverse-transcribed into cDNA, and by means of labeling this cDNA from different sources (i.e., normal cells and tumor cells) with different fluorochromes, the differential expression of distinct sets of genes can be measured. By scanning with a laser, different spots can have different colors depending on the success of binding by the two different cDNAs. This "in silica" analysis has great potential in fields such as clinical diagnosis of lymphoid tumors.

Figure 9-8. Complement fixation assay. In the complement fixation assay, complement components bind to antibody-antigen complexes, thereby making complement unavailable for hemolysis of indicator red blood cells. In the absence of specific antibody-antigen interactions, complement assembly results in cell lysis.

ABO Blood Groups and Rh Incompatibility

The ABO blood groups were first identified in 1901. They represent important antigens to be accounted for to assure safe blood transfusions (Fig. 9-10). The ABO antigens represent carbohydrate moieties present on erythrocytes. Individuals naturally develop antibodies (called isoantibodies) specific for ABO antigens that they do not express. If the individual receives a transfusion of blood that contains noncompatible ABO antigens, isoantibodies will cause agglutination of the donor cells. This process is referred to as isohemagglutination; the antigens are sometimes called *isohemagglutinins.*

Rh antigens, also called *Rhesus antigens*, are transmembrane proteins expressed at the surface of erythrocytes. They appear to be used for the transport of CO_2 and/or ammonia across the plasma membrane. Red blood cells that

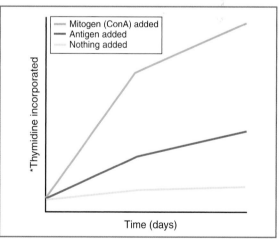

Figure 9-9. Blast transformation assay. Blast transformation assays are useful to measure cell reactivity of lymphocytes. Peripheral blood lymphocytes are incubated in the presence of mitogen or specific antigen. If reactive, lymphocytes begin to proliferate. Historically, radioactive nucleotides (^{3}H-thymidine) were added; the amount of radioactivity incorporated into DNA was determined as a quantitative measure of proliferation. The reduction of tetrazolium salts is now recognized as a safer and accurate alternative to radiometric testing. The yellow tetrazolium salt (MTT) is reduced in metabolically active cells to form insoluble purple formazan crystals, which are solubilized by the addition of a detergent. The color can then be quantified by spectrophotometric means.

Blood Group	Erythrocyte Antigens	Serum Antibodies	Genotypes
A	A	Anti-B	AA or AO
B	B	Anti-A	BB or BO
AB	A and B	Neither	AB
O	Neither	Anti-A and anti-B	OO

O Antigen	A Antigen	B Antigen

Figure 9-10. ABO phenotypes (blood groups) present in the human population and structure of terminal sugar antigenic epitopes. The blood groups represent carbohydrate antigens present on red blood cells. Antibodies specific for ABO antigens are present only if the individual does not express those determinants.

are Rh positive express the one designated D (RhD antigen). About 15% of the population have no RhD antigens and thus are "Rh negative." Of great clinical importance is the complication of RhD incompatibility between mother and fetus. An Rh-negative mother who carries an Rh-positive fetus runs the risk of producing immune antibodies to the Rh antigens on the fetal RBC. The exposure during the primary pregnancy is minimized. However, the mother may generate Rh antibodies after giving birth if she comes into contact with fetal blood cells during placental rupture. Some fetal RBCs enter the mother's bloodstream, thereby allowing production of maternal derived anti-Rh antibodies. In subsequent pregnancies, the next Rh-positive fetus will be at risk, since the mother will retain a low level of circulating antibodies against the Rh antigen. Destruction of fetal erythrocytes will ensue by passive immune transfer of maternal antibodies to fetus, resulting in erythroblastosis fetalis (hemolytic disease of the newborn). It is of great clinical importance to identify

the Rh-mismatched mother and fetus; typically, an indirect Coombs' test is performed to identify isohemagglutination. If it is positive, the mother is clinically treated with anti-Rh antibodies (Rh immune globulin [RhIG] or *RhoGAM*), which reacts with fetal RBCs. Ensuing antibody-antigen complexes are removed prior to maternal recognition of foreign Rh antigen.

KEY POINTS ABOUT IMMUNOASSAYS

- Immune experimental systems allow diagnostic assessment of infection and pathogenic responses.
- Interactions of antibodies with antigens form the basis of many qualitative and quantitative diagnostic assays.
- The affinity of the antibody-antigen reaction can be defined through physical laws of mass action.

Infection and Immunity 10

●●● MAJOR IMMUNE DEFENSE MECHANISMS AGAINST PATHOGENS

The course of response against typical acute infections can be subdivided into distinct stages. Initially, the level of infectious agent is low, beginning with breach of a mechanical barrier (e.g., skin, mucosal surface). Once inside the host, the pathogen encounters a microenvironment for suitable replication. The agent replicates, releasing antigens that trigger innate immune function, generally characterized as nonspecific. Preformed effector molecules recognize microorganisms within the first 4 hours of infection and assist in limiting expansion of the organism. Complement components and released chemokines attract professional phagocytes (macrophages and polymorphonuclear [PMN] cells) and natural killer (NK) cells to the site of infection, to assist in activation of these cells. After 4 or 5 days, antigen-specific lymphocytes (B and T cells) undergo clonal expansion, enabling directed control and eventual clearance of the infectious agent. As the agent is cleared, the host is left with residual effector cells and antibodies as well as immunologic memory to provide lasting protection against reinfection.

A wide variety of pathogenic microorganisms exist. They may be globally classified into groups: bacterial, mycobacterial, viral, protozoal, parasitic worms, and fungal. The major immune defense mechanisms are summarized in Table 10-1.

The host defense is based upon availability of resources to combat a localized pathogen (Fig. 10-1). Virtually all pathogens have an extracellular phase during which they are vulnerable to antibody-mediated effector mechanisms. An extracellular agent may reside on epithelial cell surfaces, where antibodies (immunoglobulin A [IgA]) and nonspecific inflammatory cells may be sufficient for combating infection. If the agent resides within interstitial spaces, in blood, or in lymph, then protection may also include complement components and macrophage phagocytosis and neutralization responses. Intracellular agents require a different response to be effective. For cytoplasmic agents, T lymphocytes and NK cells, as well as T-cell dependent macrophage activation, are usually necessary to kill the organism.

Pathogens can damage host tissue by direct and indirect mechanisms. Organisms may directly damage tissue by release of exotoxins that act on the surface of host cells or via released endotoxins that trigger local production of damaging cytokines. Pathogens may also directly destroy the cells they infect. Indirect damage can also occur through actions of the adaptive immune response. Pathologic damage may occur from excess deposition of antibody-antigen complexes or through bystander killing effects during overactive specific responses to infected host target cells.

Bacterial Infections

Bacterial infections begin with a breach of a mechanical barrier. Release of bacterial factors upon replication initiates a cascade of events (Fig. 10-2). Initially, infection may be resisted by antibody-mediated immune mechanisms, including neutralization of bacterial toxins. With the help of

TABLE 10-1. Major Immune Defense Mechanisms against Pathogens

Type of Infection	Major Immune Defense Mechanisms
Bacterial	Antibody, immunocomplex, and cytotoxicity
Mycobacterial	DTH and granulomatous reactions
Viral	Antibody (neutralization), CTL, and T_{DTH}
Protozoal	DTH and antibody
Parasitic worms	Antibody (atopic, ADCC) and granulomatous reactions
Fungal	DTH and granulomatous reactions

ADCC, antibody-dependent cell-mediated cytotoxicity; CTL, cytotoxic T lymphocyte; DTH, delayed-type hypersensitivity.

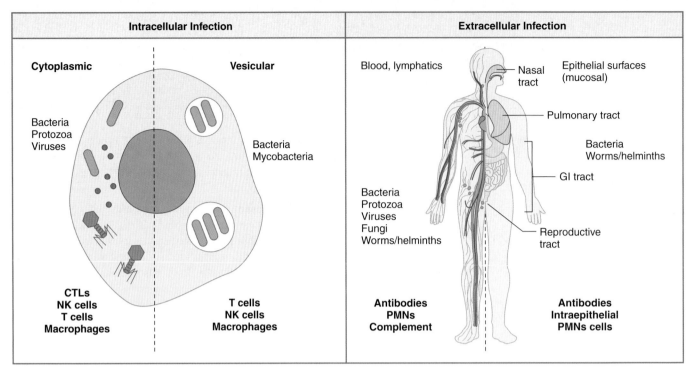

Figure 10-1. Functional immune response is dependent on organism location within the host. Effective immune responses are directed against intracellular organisms residing in cytoplasmic or vesicular space, or against extracellular organisms residing at mucosal surfaces or present in blood, lymph, or tissue.

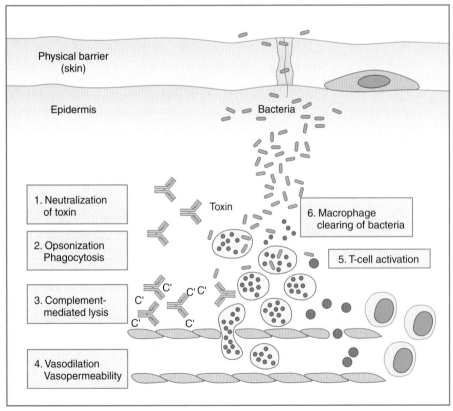

Figure 10-2. Bacterial infections. Immune defenses against bacterial agents include antibodies for neutralization of toxins, opsonization of organisms for targeted destruction, and activation of complement for direct lysis. Vasodilation of blood vessels allows entry of PMNs, macrophages, and T cells to sites of infection to assist in control of infection.

complement factors, direct cytotoxic lysis of microorganisms can occur. Release of C3a and C5a in the complement cascade causes vasodilatation and vasopermeability, resulting in an influx of professional phagocytes and acute polymorphonuclear infiltrates. Opsonization of bacteria leads to increased phagocytosis and acute anaphylactic vascular events that permit exudation of inflammatory cells and fluids. Phagocytosis may also occur via specific surface receptors for ligands such as mannose or sialic acids (pattern recognition receptors). During the chronic stage of the infection, cell-mediated immunity is activated. T cells reacting with bacterial antigens may infiltrate the site of infection, become activated, and release lymphokines that further attract and activate macrophages. Likewise, NK cells enter the infected region and assist in macrophage activation. The activated macrophages phagocytose and degrade necrotic bacteria and tissue, preparing the lesion for healing. PMNs, especially neutrophils, are an excellent example of the first line of innate defense against bacterial agents. Pus is composed of dead and dying PMN and host cells, local fluids and exudates, and dead and dying bacteria.

The role of complement in response to bacterial infection must be stressed. Major biological components of the complement system include activation of phagocytes, direct cytolysis of target cells, and opsonization of microorganisms and immunocomplexes for cells expressing complement receptors.

Important factors released by macrophages in response to bacterial antigens include cytokines that exert both local

PHARMACOLOGY

Pharmacologic Control of Inflammation

Pharmacologic control of inflammation may be managed through the use of nonsteroidal anti-inflammatory drugs (NSAIDs) or corticosteroid hormone analogs (such as prednisone). The NSAIDs as a group function as nonselective inhibitors of cyclooxygenase-1 (COX-1) and cyclooxygenase-2 (COX-2), which catalyzes the formation of prostaglandins and thromboxane from arachidonic acid.

and systemic function. Locally, IL-1, TNF-α, and IL-8 cause inflammation and activate vascular endothelial cells to increase permeability and allow more immune cells to enter infected area. TNF-α will also destroy local tissue to limit growth of bacteria. In addition, IL-6 can stimulate an increase in B-cell maturation and antibody production, and IL-12 will lead to activation of NK cells and priming of T cells toward a T_H1 response. Systemically, IL-1α, IL-1β, TNF-α, IL-6, and IL-8 all contribute to elevated body temperature (fever) and production of acute-phase proteins.

Mycobacterial Infections

Mycobacterial infections such as tuberculosis and leprosy are extremely complex (Fig. 10-3). Mycobacteria have evolved to inhibit normal macrophage killing mechanisms (e.g., phagosome-lysosome fusion) and survive within the

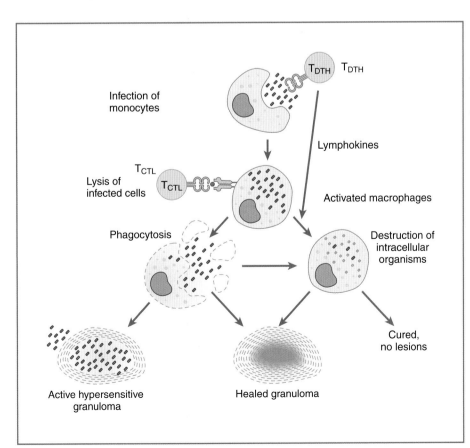

Figure 10-3. Mycobacterial infections. Immunity against mycobacteria is initiated by phagocytic macrophages, the preferred host for the infectious agent. The overall outcome and associated pathologies are dependent upon level of activation by cellular (T_{DTH}) response.

"disarmed" professional phagocyte. T_{DTH}-initiated cellular responses are the main mechanisms involved in an active immune response, including granulomatous hypersensitivity, but only after infection has become established. Both helper and cytotoxic T cells are responsible for control and containment of active infection. They recognize mycobacterial antigens and glycolipids presented on the surface of infected cells, leading to release of cytokines and chemokines that recruit additional immune effectors. A local environment is established to contain infection, resulting in granuloma pathology. Healing of the infected center may occur, with limited necrosis of the infected tissue. If the infection persists, an active caseous granuloma may form with a necrotic nidus composed of infected and active macrophages. The granuloma is usually circumscribed by responding T cells, with host-mediated destructive response occurring inside the area of organism containment. The presence of giant cells (activated syncytial multinucleated epithelioid cells) is characteristic of late-stage response.

At one time it was thought that the tissue lesions of tuberculosis required the effect of delayed-type hypersensitivity. The term *hypersensitivity* was coined because animals with cellular immune reactivity to tubercle bacilli developed greater tissue lesions after reinoculation of bacilli than did animals injected for the first time. The granulomatous lesions seen in tuberculosis depend upon primary innate functions as well as acquired immune mechanisms; lesions are not the cause of disease but an unfortunate effect of protective mechanisms. In the lung, extensive damage with accompanying caseous granulomatous pathology can ultimately result in respiratory failure. The granulomatous immune response produces the lesion, but the mycobacterium causes the disease.

Viral Infections

Immune responses to viral agents are dependent upon location of the virus within the host (Fig. 10-4). Antibodies play a critical role during the extracellular life cycle of the virus. Antibodies can bind to virus-forming complexes that can inactivate virions and allow them to be cleared effectively by professional phagocytes. Humoral responses can prevent the entry of virus particles into cells by interfering with the

ability of the virus to attach to a host cell, and secretory IgA can prevent the establishment of viral infections of mucous membranes. Once viral infection is established within cells, it is no longer susceptible to the effects of antibody. Upon entry to cells, immune resistance to viral infections is primarily T cell–mediated. To be effective in attacking intracellular organisms, an immune mechanism must have the capacity to react with cells in solid tissue. This is a property of cell-mediated reactions—particularly with cytotoxic T lymphocytes (CTLs)—but not of antibody-mediated reactions.

Most nucleated cells have an inherent, but limited, mechanism to down-regulate viral replication through self-production of IFN-α and IFN-β. However, these nonspecific interferon responses are not sufficient to eliminate the virus. NK cells are an early component of the host response to viral infection. NK cells nonspecifically recognize and kill virally infected targets. NK cells provide a link between innate and adaptive immunity, since they produce multiple immunomodulatory cytokines (e.g., IFN-γ, TNF-α, transforming growth factor-β [TGF-β] and IL-10). In addition, NK cells release IFN-γ (physically different from the other interferons) and IL-12, molecules that both activate macrophages and help prime T cells for an effective antiviral T_H1 response.

Virus-infected cells will at some stage of the infection express viral antigens on the cell surface in combination with class I molecules. Specific sensitized CD8$^+$ CTL cells recognize presented viral antigens and destroy virus-infected cells (and therefore limit viral replication) through release of factors that include granzymes, perforins, and interferons. Lethal signals may be delivered through Fas/Fas-ligand–mediated mechanisms. Adverse effects occur if the cell expressing the viral antigens is important functionally, as is the case for certain viral infections of the central nervous system. If the virus-infected target is a macrophage, lymphocyte T_H cells exhibiting delayed-type hypersensitivity (T_{DTH}) can activate the macrophages to kill their intracellular viruses; lymphokine-activated macrophages produce a variety of enzymes and cytokines that can inactivate viruses. The critical nature of T cell–mediated response to viral infections is evident in patients whose cell-mediated immunity (CMI) is defective.

Parasitic Infections (Helminths)

Host responses to parasitic worm infections are generally more complex because the pathogen is larger and not able to be engulfed by phagocytes (Fig. 10-5). Helminths typically undergo life cycle changes as they adapt for life in the host. Worms are located in the intestinal tract or tissues. Tapeworms, which exist in only the intestinal lumen, promote no protective immunologic response. On the other hand, worms with larval forms that invade tissue typically stimulate an immune response. The tissue reaction to *Ascaris* and *Trichinella* consists of an intense infiltrate of polymorphonuclear leukocytes, with a predominance of eosinophils. Therefore, a variety of antigens that are life cycle stage–dependent are displayed in changing tissue environments. Numerous

---

PATHOLOGY

Granulomatous Response to *Mycobacterium tuberculosis*

Cell-mediated response to mycobacterial antigens results in disruption of normal pulmonary architecture and development of a granulomatous response. Late-stage disease is characterized by large granulomas with central caseation, a process of necrosis that includes elements of liquefactive and coagulative necrosis. Cavities near the lung apex can allow entry of liquefied necrotic material into eroded airways, leading to spread of infectious agents via aerosolization.

Figure 10-4. Viral infections. Immunity against viral infections is threefold, with contributions by antibodies, cytotoxic T cells, and T$_H$ cells.

Antibody to virus
Binds to viral receptors and blocks attachment to cell

Class I
CD8$^+$ T$_{CTL}$ reacts with viral antigens on surface of infected cell, perforin release causes lysis of infected cells

Class II
CD4$^+$ T$_{DTH}$ reacts with viral antigens on surface of infected cell, lymphokines attract and activate phagocytosis by macrophages

cells play a role, depending on the location of the organism. Antigens on the surface of organisms or released into the local environment may stimulate T cells and macrophages to interact with B cells to secrete specific antibodies. IL-5, a T cell–derived factor, is instrumental in stimulation of eosinophils; the eosinophils act by associating with specific antibody to kill worms by antibody-dependent cell-mediated cytotoxicity (ADCC) or by releasing enzymes from granules to exert controlling effects on mast cells.

Antigen reacting with IgE antibody bound to intestinal mast cells stimulates release of inflammatory mediators, such as histamine, proteases, leukotrienes, prostaglandins, and serotonin. These agents cause an increase in the vascular permeability of the mucosa, exposing worms to serum immune components, and stimulate increased mucus production and increased peristalsis. These activities are associated with expulsion of parasitic worms from the gastrointestinal tract through formation of a physical barrier to limit adherence and interactions with the mucosal surface.

Eosinophil granules contain basic proteins that are toxic to worms. Eosinophils may be directed to attack helminths by cytophilic antibodies that bridge the eosinophil through the Fc region and the helminth by specific Fab-binding ADCC. Anaphylactic antibodies (IgE) are frequently associated with helminth infections, and intradermal injection of worm extracts elicits wheal-and-flare reactions. Children infested with *Ascaris lumbricoides* have attacks of urticaria, asthma, and other anaphylactic or atopic reactions presumably associated with dissemination of *Ascaris* antigens.

PATHOLOGY

Urticaria

Urticaria, or hives, resulting from localized mast cell degranulation, are wheal-and-flare reactions on the skin surface, with accompanying angioedema in deeper layers of the dermis.

Fungal Infections

Relatively little is known about the immune response to fungal agents. Cellular immunity appears to be the most important immunologic factor in resistance to fungal infections, although humoral antibody certainly may play a role. T$_H$1 type responses are protective via release of IFN-γ. By contrast, T$_H$2 responses (IL-4 and IL-10) typically correlate with disease exacerbation and pathology. The importance of cellular reactions is indicated by the intense mononuclear infiltrate and granulomatous reactions that occur in tissues infected with fungi and by the fact that fungal infections are frequently associated with depressed immune reactivity of the delayed type (opportunistic infections). For example, the condition of chronic mucocutaneous candidiasis caused by persistent or recurrent infection by *Candida albicans* usually manifests only in patients with general depression of cellular immune reactions. As a general rule, fungi appear to be resistant to the effects of antibody, and CMI is needed for effective resistance.

Figure 10-5. Response to parasitic worms. Immune activity against parasitic worms is directed by T_H2 cells, driving activation of eosinophils, basophils, and mast cells to release inflammatory mediators to limit parasitic activity and kill invading organisms.

Parasitic antigens

Macrophage

T_H2 cell

B cell

GM-CSF
IL-3

IL-4
IL-5

IL-4
IL-6

IgE, Fc cross-link receptor

Eosinophil activation

Degranulation

Mast cell/ basophil activation

- Eosinophil cationic protein
- Eosinophil-derived neurotoxin
- Major basic protein
- Eosinophil peroxidase
- Eosinophil collagenase
- Leukotrienes
- Platelet-activating factor

- Histamines
- Tryptase, cathepsin G
- IL-3, IL-5, GM-CSF (promotes eosinophil activation)
- IL-4, IL-13 (promotes T_H2 response)
- Leukotrienes
- Platelet-activating factor

KEY POINTS ABOUT MAJOR IMMUNE DEFENSE MECHANISMS AGAINST PATHOGENS

- The host defense is based upon availability of resources to combat a localized pathogen.
- Virtually all pathogens have an extracellular phase during which they are vulnerable to antibody-mediated effector mechanisms and complement components, macrophage phagocytosis, and neutralization responses.
- Intracellular agents usually require T lymphocytes (helper and cytotoxic) and NK cells, as well as T cell–dependent macrophage activation, to kill organisms.
- Pathogens can damage host tissue by direct and indirect mechanisms.
- The main immune mechanisms against pathogens are *bacterial,* antibody (immunocomplex and cytotoxicity); *mycobacterial,* DTH and granulomatous reactions; *viral,* antibody (neutralization), CTL, and T_{DTH}; *protozoal,* DTH and antibody; *parasitic worms,* antibody (atopic, ADCC) and granulomatous reactions; *fungal,* DTH and granulomatous reactions.

●●● IMMUNE DEVIATION: DOMINANCE OF ONE RESPONSE OVER ANOTHER

Immune deviation, or split tolerance, is defined as the dominance of one immune response mechanism over another for a specific antigen and has been implicated in the tendency for certain individuals to develop IgE (allergic) antibodies rather than IgG antibodies. In addition, for reasons that may be genetically determined, some individuals tend to make strong cellular immune responses but weak antibody response to certain antigens, whereas other individuals will have the opposite responses.

The biological function of granulomatous reactivity is exemplified by the spectrum of pathology presented during infection with *Mycobacterium leprae,* the causative agent for leprosy. The clinical manifestations of leprosy are determined by the immune response of the patient. Leprosy is classified into three major overlapping groups: tuberculoid, borderline, and lepromatous. Tuberculoid leprosy is associated with delayed hypersensitivity and the formation of prominent, well-formed granulomatous lesions, many lymphocytes, and few if any organisms. Delayed hypersensitivity skin tests are intact, and there is predominant hyperplasia of the diffuse cortex (T-cell zone) of the lymph nodes. The low resistance characteristic of lepromatous leprosy is associated with the accumulation of "foamy" macrophages filled with viable organisms and the presence of high levels of humoral antibodies. Delayed hypersensitivity skin tests are depressed, and there is marked follicular hyperplasia in the lymph nodes with little or no diffuse cortex. The levels of antibodies are high, and vascular lesions due to immunocomplexes are seen (erythema nodosum leprosum). Borderline leprosy has intermediate findings.

This example of the forms of leprosy illustrates both the role of cellular immunity (delayed hypersensitivity) in controlling the infection and the lack of protective response provided by humoral antibodies. The cytokine patterns in the two polar forms of the disease are different. Typically T_H2 cytokines (IL-4, IL-5, and IL-10) dominate in the lepromatous form, whereas cytokines produced by T_H1 cells (IFN-γ, TNF, and IL-2) predominate in tuberculoid leprosy. IFN-γ would be expected to activate macrophages to kill intracellular pathogens and control organism expansion; high IL-4 may explain hypergammaglobulinemia in lepromatous patients. A diagram illustrating the relationship of the degree of cellular and humoral immune response to the stages of leprosy is shown (Fig. 10-6).

KEY POINTS ABOUT IMMUNE DEVIATION

- The response to initial infection is divided into phases.
- The first phase is an early innate and nonspecific response, in which preformed effector cells and molecules recognize microorganisms.
- The next phase is again primarily a nonspecific encounter with the organism, characterized by recruitment of professional phagocytes and NK cells to the site of infection.

- The final phase involves antigen-specific cell (B and T lymphocyte) effectors that undergo clonal expansion; these cells provide memory responses in case of reinfection.

●●● EVASION OF IMMUNE RESPONSE

In the ongoing evolution of host-parasite relationships between humans and their infections, infectious organisms have developed "ingenious" ways to avoid immune defense mechanisms (Table 10-2). Organisms may locate in niches (privileged sites) not accessible to immune effector mechanisms (*protective niche*) or hide themselves by acquiring host molecules (*masking*). They may change their surface antigens (*antigenic modulation*), hide within cells, and produce factors that inhibit the immune response

TABLE 10-2. Pathogen Evasion of Immune Response

Mechanisms	Examples
Localization in protective niches	Latent syphilis, tapeworm (*Echinococcus*)
Intracellular location	Histoplasmosis, herpesvirus, varicella, HIV
Antigenic modulation	Malaria, trypanosomiasis, relapsing fever
Preservation of receptor sites after reaction with antibody	Influenza virus
Immunosuppression	Malaria, measles, HIV, tuberculosis (anergy)
Inappropriate immune response (immune deviation)	Lepromatous leprosy, chronic mucocutaneous candidiasis

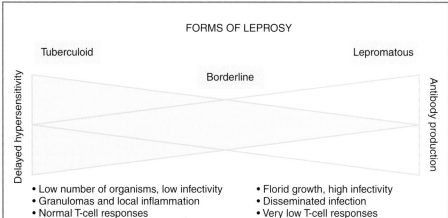

FORMS OF LEPROSY

Tuberculoid   Lepromatous

Borderline

Delayed hypersensitivity   Antibody production

- Low number of organisms, low infectivity
- Granulomas and local inflammation
- Normal T-cell responses
- T_H1 cytokines: IFN-γ, TNF-α, and IL-2)

- Florid growth, high infectivity
- Disseminated infection
- Very low T-cell responses
- T_H2 cytokines: IL-4, IL-5, and IL-10

Figure 10-6. Immune deviation in response to *Mycobacterium leprae*. The overlapping triangles indicate the relative strength of delayed hypersensitivity and antibody production. The solid triangle indicates delayed hypersensitivity; the open triangle, antibody production. High levels of delayed-type hypersensitivity (DTH) are associated with cure of tuberculoid leprosy; weak DTH is associated with progressive disease; balanced DTH and antibody production with borderline leprosy and slowly progressive disease.

(*immunosuppression*) or fool the immune system into responding with an ineffective effector mechanism (*immune deviation*). The ultimate endpoint of coevolution of the human host and its infectious organisms results in an eventual mutual coexistence with most environmental organisms. No better evidence is the loss of this coexistence when the immune mechanisms do not function properly. Then, organisms that do not normally cause disease become virulent. The lesson of AIDS (infection with the human immunodeficiency virus [HIV]) demonstrates that opportunistic infectious organisms will become dominant when introduced into a previously unexposed population. In a fully evolved, mature relationship, host and infectious agent initially coexist with limited detrimental affects. Thus, the ultimate evolution of the host parasite relationship is not "cure" of an infection by complete elimination of the parasite, but at least mutual coexistence without deleterious effects of the parasite on the host. In fact, in many human infections, the infectious agent is never fully destroyed and the disease enters a latent state, only to be reactivated when immune surveillance wanes. For example, 70% of the population has been exposed to cytomegalovirus; transplant patients who are therapeutically immunosuppressed are at much greater risk for development of infection-related disease.

Bacteria have evolved to evade different aspects of phagocyte-mediated killing (Fig. 10-7). For example, they may (1) secrete toxins to inhibit chemotaxis, (2) contain outer capsules that block attachment, (3) block intracellular fusion with lysosomal compartments, and (4) escape from the phagosome to multiply in the cytoplasm. Viral entities also subvert immune responses, usually through the presence of virally encoded proteins. Some of these proteins block effector functions of antibody binding, block complement-mediated pathways, inhibit activation of infected cells, and can down-regulate MHC class I antigens to escape CTL killing. Herpesvirus produces a factor that inhibits inflammatory responses by blocking effects of cytokines through receptor mimicking, and another that blocks proper antigen presentation and processing. Finally, Epstein-Barr virus encodes a cytokine homolog of IL-10 that leads to immunosuppression of the host by activating T_H2 rather than T_H1 responses.

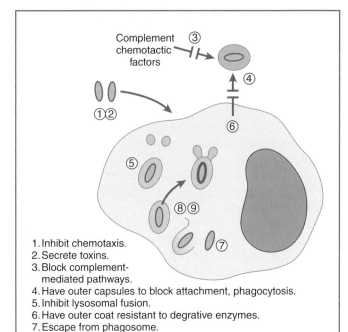

1. Inhibit chemotaxis.
2. Secrete toxins.
3. Block complement-mediated pathways.
4. Have outer capsules to block attachment, phagocytosis.
5. Inhibit lysosomal fusion.
6. Have outer coat resistant to degrative enzymes.
7. Escape from phagosome.
8. Turn off cytokine activation.
9. Activate cytokines inappropriately.

Figure 10-7. Mechanisms of infectious organisms to avoid immune defenses. Organisms evade immune responses through various mechanisms including location in protective niches, acquisition of host molecules, alteration of surface antigens, and producing factors to inhibit or redirect effective immune response.

KEY POINTS ABOUT EVASION OF IMMUNE RESPONSE

- Virtually all classes of infectious agents have devised ways to avoid host defenses.
- Mechanisms include inaccessibility in protective niches, antigenic modulation of surface molecules, and release of factors to either suppress the immune response or cause immune deviation and ineffective response to the agent.

SECTION II

Microbiology

Basic Bacteriology 11

At least 800 different species of bacteria inhabit the human host, representing a total population approaching 10^{15} organisms. Put into perspective, the number of bacteria is far greater than the number of cells in our bodies. Many organisms colonize various body tissues, representing specific flora that take advantage of space and nutrients in a commensal existence. However, organisms that forgo commensal or symbiotic relationships can produce disease and pathogenic response.

●●● BACTERIAL STRUCTURE, FUNCTION, AND CLASSIFICATION

Historically, organisms were classified according to physical parameters, such as microscopic morphology (size and shape), staining characteristics, and ability to multiply on various energy sources (Fig. 11-1). Identification of specific biomarkers (biotyping) allowed classification for epidemiologic purposes, identifying organisms according to metabolic activity due to presence or absence of enzymes or ability to grow on specific substrates. The advent of antibiotics allowed further classification according to drug susceptibility patterns; and antibody-based serotyping was used to determine specific antigenic surface molecules unique to groups of bacterial organisms.

Recent development of molecular biological tools has led to genotypic classification with greater precision than that of past methodologies. Genetic characterization of organisms is based directly on nucleic acid sequence and DNA homology, on nucleotide content (ratios of guanine plus cytosine), on analysis of plasmid content, or on ribotyping (RNA complement of a cell).

KEY POINTS ABOUT BACTERIAL STRUCTURE, FUNCTION, AND CLASSIFICATION

- Bacteria are classified according to morphologic structure, metabolic activity, and environmental factors needed for survival.
- Gram-positive organisms are so named because of staining characteristics inherent in their thick peptidoglycan outer layer with teichoic and lipoteichoic acid present; gram-negative bacteria have a thin peptidoglycan component surrounding a periplasmic space, as well as an outer membrane with associated lipoproteins.
- Other bacterial species, such as the mycobacteria, have unique glycolipids that give them a waxy appearance and unique biological advantages during infection of the host.

●●● GENERAL PROPERTIES OF PROKARYOTIC ORGANISMS

Prokaryotic organisms have distinct characteristics from eukaryotes. Prokaryotic cells do not have a nuclear membrane; instead, their haploid circular DNA is loosely

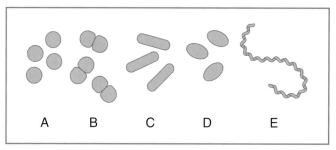

Figure 11-1. Bacterial morphologies. The diverse morphology of bacteria is related to physical characteristics of the outer cell membrane. Some of the diverse bacterial forms are cocci (**A**), diplococci (**B**), bacilli (**C**), coccobacilli (**D**), and spirochetes (**E**).

organized as a fibrous mass in the cytoplasm. Bacteria do not have organelles, unique Golgi apparatus, or true endoplasmic reticulum; rather, transcription and translation are coupled events. Bacterial 70S ribosomes, consisting of 30S and 50S subunits, are significantly different from eukaryotic 80S ribosomes, thus allowing potential targets for antimicrobials.

The cell envelope surrounding a bacterium includes a cell membrane and a peptidoglycan layer. Two major classes of bacteria are distinguishable by staining patterns following exposure to primary stain, gram iodine, and alcohol decolorization. *Gram-positive organisms* maintain a purple color from the primary stain incorporated into the thick peptidoglycan layer that surrounds the organism (Fig. 11-2). *Gram-negative organisms* have a reduced peptidoglycan layer surrounded by an outer membrane. The peptidoglycan layer is a complex polymer composed of alternating N-acetylglucosamine and N-acetylmuramic acid with attached tetrapeptide side chains. The bonds linking the N-acetylglucosamine and N-acetylmuramic acid are especially sensitive to cleavage by lysozyme, commonly found in saliva, tears, and mucosal secretions (useful basic host defense

mechanisms). Gram-positive cell membranes are further characterized by the presence of teichoic and teichuronic acids (water-soluble polymers) chemically bonded to the peptidoglycan layer. Gram-negative bacteria are further characterized by the presence of a periplasmic space between the cell membrane and the outer membrane. The outer membrane comprises a phospholipid bilayer with embedded proteins that assist in energy conversion (such as cytochromes and enzymes involved in electron transport and oxidative phosphorylation). The cytoplasmic membrane also contains enzymes critical for cell wall biosynthesis, phospholipid synthesis and DNA replication, and proteins that assist in transport of needed molecules.

Lipopolysaccharide (LPS) is contained within the outer membrane of gram-negative organisms and comprises polysaccharide (O) side chains, core polysaccharides, and lipid A endotoxin. Lipid A contains fatty acids that are inserted into the bacterial outer membrane. The remaining extracellular portion of LPS is free to interact with host immune cells during infection, acting as a powerful immunostimulant via binding to CD14 receptor on macrophages and endothelial

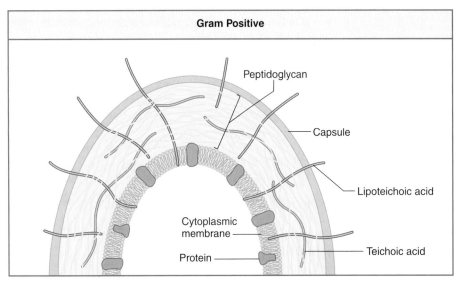

Gram Positive

- Peptidoglycan
- Capsule
- Lipoteichoic acid
- Cytoplasmic membrane
- Protein
- Teichoic acid

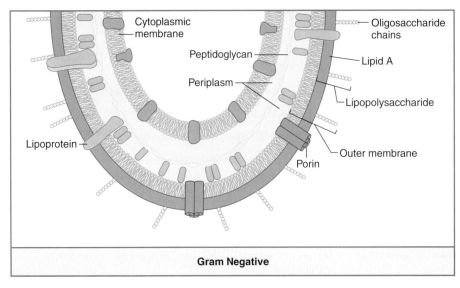

- Cytoplasmic membrane
- Peptidoglycan
- Periplasm
- Lipoprotein
- Porin
- Oligosaccharide chains
- Lipid A
- Lipopolysaccharide
- Outer membrane

Gram Negative

Figure 11-2. Gram-positive and gram-negative cell walls. The gram-positive bacteria have a characteristic thick peptidoglycan layer surrounding an inner cytoplasmic membrane. The gram-negative bacteria have reduced peptidoglycan surrounded by periplasm, with an outer membrane comprising embedded core lipopolysaccharide and lipid A endotoxin. Both gram-positive and gram-negative bacteria may also support an outer glycocalyx or capsule (not depicted). Upon treatment with gram iodine, gram-positive bacteria resist alcohol treatment and retain stain, whereas gram-negative organisms can be differentiated by loss of the primary stain and later addition of a safranin counterstain.

cells, resulting in secretion of interleukins, chemokines, and inflammatory cytokines. Lipid core polysaccharides contain ketodeoxyoctonate (KDO) as well as other sugars (e.g., ketodeoxyoctulonate and heptulose) and two glucosamine sugar derivatives. Lipoproteins link the thin peptidoglycan layer to an outer membrane.

Certain gram-positive and -negative organisms may also have a capsule, or glycocalyx layer, external to the cell wall, containing antigenic proteins. The capsule protects bacteria from phagocytosis by monocytes and can also play a role in adherence to host tissue. The glycocalyx is a loose network of polysaccharide fibers with adhesive properties containing embedded antigenic proteins. Organisms can be characterized by the presence of appendages, such as flagella, which assist in locomotion, or pili (fimbriae), which allow adhesion to host tissue; sex pili are involved in attachment of donor and recipient organisms during replication.

●●● BACTERIAL PHYSIOLOGY

All microorganisms of medical significance require energy obtained through exothermic reactions—chemosynthesis—and all require a source of carbon. Organisms capable of using CO_2 are considered auxotrophs. Many pathogenic organisms are able to utilize complex organic compounds; however, almost all can survive on simple organic compounds such as glucose. The main scheme for producing energy is through glycolysis via the Embden-Meyerhof pathway (Fig. 11-3). Two

A

B

Figure 11-3. Energy schemes employed by bacteria. Two of the three main energy producing schemes employed by bacteria for production of energy are the Embden-Meyerhof pathway (glycolysis) (**A**) and utilization of pyruvate through the tricarboxylic acid (TCA) cycle to produce NADH, $FADH_2$, and ATP (**B**). A third method (not shown) utilizes oxidative phosphorylation through the electron transport chain.

other main sources for energy production are the tricarbo-xylic acid (TCA) cycle and oxidative phosphorylation. Alternatively, the pentose-phosphate pathway may be used.

Facultative organisms can live under aerobic or anaerobic conditions. Obligate aerobes are restricted to the use of oxygen as the final electron acceptor. Anaerobes (growing in the absence of molecular O_2) use the process of fermentation, which may be defined as the energy-yielding anaerobic metabolic breakdown of a nutrient molecule, such as glucose, without net oxidation. Fermentation yields lactate, acetic acid, ethanol, or other simple products (e.g., formic acid).

Many bacteria are saprophytes, growing on decayed animal or vegetable matter. Saprophytes do not normally invade living tissue, but rather grow in our environment. However, saprophytic organisms can become pathogenic in immuno-suppressed individuals or in devitalized tissue, as seen with species of *Clostridium*.

KEY POINTS ABOUT BACTERIAL PHYSIOLOGY

- The three main schemes for producing energy in bacteria are glycolysis, the TCA cycle, and oxidative phosphorylation.
- Alternative schemes are used, such as fermentation, to assist organisms growing under anaerobic conditions.

●●● COMMENSAL ORGANISMS OF THE NORMAL BODY FLORA

The body is host to a tremendous number of commensal organisms, existing in a symbiotic relationship in which a bacterial species derives benefit and the host is relatively unharmed (Fig. 11-4). The normal body flora consists of organisms that take advantage of the interface between the host and the environment, with presence of defined species on exposed surfaces as well as throughout the respiratory, gastrointestinal, and reproductive tracts. Estimates are that a normal human body houses about 10^{12} bacteria on the skin, 10^{10} in the mouth, and 10^{14} in the gastrointestinal tract—numbers far in excess of eukaryotic cells in the entire body. The interaction between human host and residing normal body flora has evolved to the benefit of the host. For example, the

normal flora prevents colonization of the body by competing pathogens and may even stimulate the production of cross-protective antibodies against invading organisms. In addition, the flora colonizing the gastrointestinal tract secretes excess vitamins (vitamins K and B_{12}), which benefit the host.

While the skin functions as a physical barrier to the outside world, it also serves as host for *Staphylococcus epidermidis* and *Corynebacteria diphtheriae*, both implicated in acne formation. The most important single mechanism for the purpose of keeping healthy is to frequently wash the hands to limit spread of both commensal and pathogenic bacteria. In the respiratory tract, nasal carriage is a primary niche for opportunistic *Staphylococcus aureus*, while the pharynx is commonly host to colonization by *Neisseria meningitidis*, *Haemophilus influenzae*, and streptococcal species. The upper respiratory tract commonly captures organisms in the mucosal layer, with subsequent clearance by cilia. The lower respiratory tract requires more aggressive methods for bacterial clearance, with heavy reliance upon macrophages and phagocytes to maintain relative balance of bacterial cell numbers.

The oral cavity and gastrointestinal tract are host to a variety of organisms with physical properties allowing commensalism in these tissues. The mouth is host to more than 300 species of bacteria, while the stomach hosts fewer numbers of organisms that can survive the acidic environment (pH ≤ 2.0). The small bowel is relatively barren of organisms owing to fast moving peristalsis, whereas the slower mobility of the large intestine allows residence of a high number of bile-resistant enteric pathogens (e.g., *Bacteroides* species), thus producing large numbers of aerobes and facultative anaerobes in the stool.

The reproductive organs are also host to a variety of organisms; *Escherichia coli* and group B streptococcus are commonly associated with vaginal epithelium, where they exist under conditions of high acidity. Indeed, *Lactobacillus acidophilus* colonizes the vaginal epithelium during child-bearing years and helps establish the low pH that inhibits the growth of other pathogens. Expansion of organisms then occurs readily in postmenopausal women, who lose general acidity of this tissue.

BIOCHEMISTRY

Pentose-Phosphate Pathway

The pentose-phosphate pathway, also called the hexose monophosphate shunt, is an alternative mode of glucose oxidation that is coupled to the formation of reduced coenzyme NADPH, giving rise to phosphogluconate. The production of biosynthetic sugars is regulated by transketolases and transaldolases. In eukaryotic cells, the phosphogluconate path is the principal source of reducing power for biosynthetic reactions in most cells.

HISTOLOGY

Respiratory Cilia

Ciliated cells throughout conducting airways continue into the respiratory tract well past mucus-producing cells, in essence preventing mucus accumulation. Goblet cells are the unicellular mucous glands, aptly named since mucus accumulation in the apical portion gives the appearance of a goblet globe and the compressed basal portion of the cytoplasm gives the appearance of a goblet stem. Mucus stains poorly with hematoxylin and eosin. The abundant concentration of goblet cells decreases progressively in the bronchial passages, and they are completely absent from terminal bronchiole epithelium.

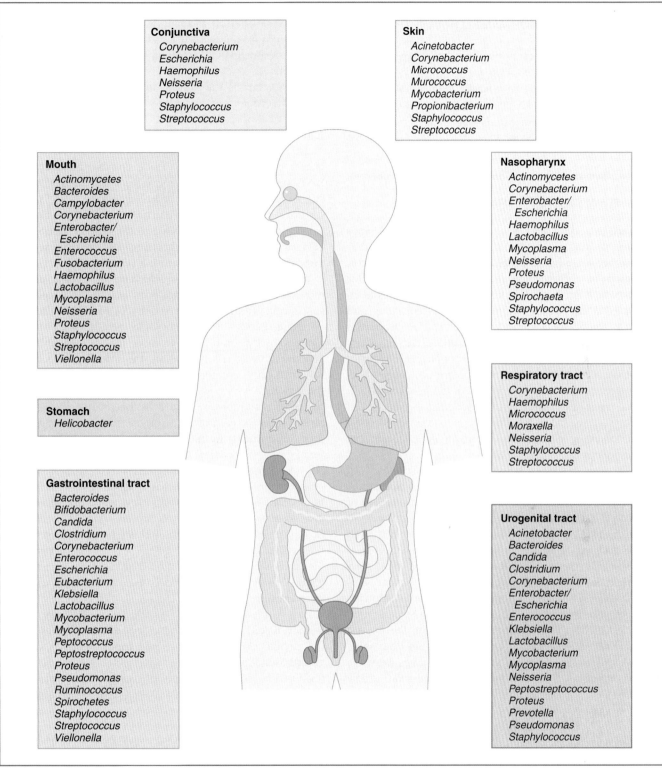

Conjunctiva
- *Corynebacterium*
- *Escherichia*
- *Haemophilus*
- *Neisseria*
- *Proteus*
- *Staphylococcus*
- *Streptococcus*

Skin
- *Acinetobacter*
- *Corynebacterium*
- *Micrococcus*
- *Murococcus*
- *Mycobacterium*
- *Propionibacterium*
- *Staphylococcus*
- *Streptococcus*

Mouth
- *Actinomycetes*
- *Bacteroides*
- *Campylobacter*
- *Corynebacterium*
- *Enterobacter/ Escherichia*
- *Enterococcus*
- *Fusobacterium*
- *Haemophilus*
- *Lactobacillus*
- *Mycoplasma*
- *Neisseria*
- *Proteus*
- *Staphylococcus*
- *Streptococcus*
- *Viellonella*

Nasopharynx
- *Actinomycetes*
- *Corynebacterium*
- *Enterobacter/ Escherichia*
- *Haemophilus*
- *Lactobacillus*
- *Mycoplasma*
- *Neisseria*
- *Proteus*
- *Pseudomonas*
- *Spirochaeta*
- *Staphylococcus*
- *Streptococcus*

Respiratory tract
- *Corynebacterium*
- *Haemophilus*
- *Micrococcus*
- *Moraxella*
- *Neisseria*
- *Staphylococcus*
- *Streptococcus*

Stomach
- *Helicobacter*

Gastrointestinal tract
- *Bacteroides*
- *Bifidobacterium*
- *Candida*
- *Clostridium*
- *Corynebacterium*
- *Enterococcus*
- *Escherichia*
- *Eubacterium*
- *Klebsiella*
- *Lactobacillus*
- *Mycobacterium*
- *Mycoplasma*
- *Peptococcus*
- *Peptostreptococcus*
- *Proteus*
- *Pseudomonas*
- *Ruminococcus*
- *Spirochetes*
- *Staphylococcus*
- *Streptococcus*
- *Viellonella*

Urogenital tract
- *Acinetobacter*
- *Bacteroides*
- *Candida*
- *Clostridium*
- *Corynebacterium*
- *Enterobacter/ Escherichia*
- *Enterococcus*
- *Klebsiella*
- *Lactobacillus*
- *Mycobacterium*
- *Mycoplasma*
- *Neisseria*
- *Peptostreptococcus*
- *Proteus*
- *Prevotella*
- *Pseudomonas*
- *Staphylococcus*

Figure 11-4. Tissue tropisms for commensal bacterial flora. The normal body flora represents organisms with tropism for specific anatomic sites. While internal tissues remain relatively free of bacterial species, tissue that is in contact with the environment, whether directly or indirectly, can be readily colonized. Some of the more common bacteria associated with specific anatomic sites of the human host are listed.

BACTERIAL GENETICS

An average bacterium has a genome composed of 3000 genes contained in single double- stranded, supercoiled DNA chromosome; some bacteria contain multiple chromosomes. In addition to chromosomal DNA, bacteria may harbor plasmids, which are small, circular, nonchromosomal, double-stranded DNA molecules. Plasmids are self-replicating and frequently contain genes that confer protective properties including antibiotic resistance and virulence factors. Many bacteria also contain viruses or bacteriophages. Bacterio-phages have a protein coat that enables them to survive outside the bacterial host; upon infection of the host bacterium, the phage replicates to large numbers, sometimes causing cell lysis. Alternatively, the phage may integrate into the bacterial genome, resulting in transfer of novel genetic material between organisms.

The transfer of genes between bacterial species is a powerful tool for adaptation to changing environments. Genes may be transferred between organisms by a variety of mechanisms, including DNA sequence exchange and recombination. Transferred genes or sequences may be integrated into the bacterial genome or stably maintained as extra-chromosomal elements. If DNA sequences being transferred are similar, homologous recombination may occur. Non-homologous recombination is a more complex event allowing transfer of nonsimilar sequences, often resulting in mutation or deletion of host genomic material. Although the highest efficiency of genetic exchange occurs within the same bacterial species, mechanisms exist for exchange between different organisms, thus readily allowing acquisition of new characteristics. Since the average number of commensal bacteria in the body approaches 10^{14}, there are an enormous number of traits and variability in bacterial gene pools. It is no wonder that the incidence and acquisition of drug resistance is so high.

Methods of Genetic Transfer Between Organisms

The three main ways to transfer genes between bacterial organisms are conjugation, transduction, and transformation (Fig. 11-5).

Bacterial *conjugation* is the bacterial equivalent of sexual reproduction or mating. To perform conjugation, one bacterium has to carry a transferable plasmid (referred to as either an F+ or an R+ plasmid), while the other must not. The transfer of plasmid DNA occurs from the F-positive bacterial cell to the F-negative bacterium (making it F+ once transfer is complete).

Transduction is the process in which DNA is transferred from one bacterium to another by way of bacteriophage. When bacteriophages infect bacteria, their mode of reproduction is to utilize the DNA replication proteins and mechanisms of the host bacterial cell to make abundant copies of their own DNA. These copies of bacteriophage DNA are then packaged into virions, which have been newly synthesized. The packaging of bacteriophage DNA is subject to error, with frequent occurrences of mispackaging of small pieces of bacterial DNA into the virions instead of the bacteriophage genome. Such virions can then be spread to new bacteria upon subsequent infection.

Transformation is a way in which mobile genetic elements move around to different positions within the genome of a single cell. Transposons are sequences of DNA, also called "jumping genes" or "transposable genetic elements," that move directly from one position to another within the genome. During transformation, the insertion of sequences can both cause mutation and change the amount of DNA in the genome.

Bacteria multiply by binary fission. Figure 11-6 shows a model of bacterial growth, with growth rate directly tied to levels of nutrients in the local environment. The rate of bacterial growth is also dependent upon the specific organism; *E. coli* in nutrient broth will replicate in 20 minutes, whereas *Mycobacterium tuberculosis* has a doubling time of 28 to 34 hours. Bacterial DNA replication is a sequential three-phase process that utilizes a variety of proteins (Fig. 11-7). Initiation of replication begins at a unique genetic site, referred to as the origin of replication. Chain elongation occurs in a bidirectional mode. The addition of nucleotides occurs in the 5′ to 3′ direction; one strand is rapidly copied (the leading strand) while the other (the lagging strand) is discontinuously copied as small fragments (Okazaki pieces) that are enzymatically linked by way of ligases and DNA polymerases. As the circular chromosome unwinds, topoisomerases, or DNA gyrases, function to relax the supercoiling that occurs. Finally, termination and segregation of newly replicated genetic

GENETICS

Histones and Chromosomes

Human genetic material is complexed with histone proteins (two each of H2a, H2b, H3, and H4 and one linker H1 molecule) and organized into nucleosomes, which are further condensed into chromatin. This gives rise to the chromosome structure. Approximately 3 billion basepairs of DNA encoding 30,000 to 40,000 genes are present within the 23 pairs of tightly coiled chromosomes.

Transformation

A

Transduction

B

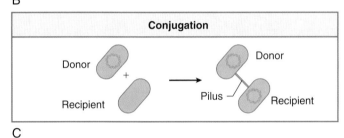

Conjugation

C

Figure 11-5. Transfer of genetic material between bacterial species through transformation, transduction, or conjugation. In transformation (**A**), naked DNA is taken up directly by recipient bacteria, sometimes mediated by surface competence factors. Transduction (**B**) utilizes bacteriophages to mediate direct transfer of nucleic acids. Conjugation (**C**) is one-way transfer of plasmids by means of physical contact, often associated with transfer of drug resistance genes.

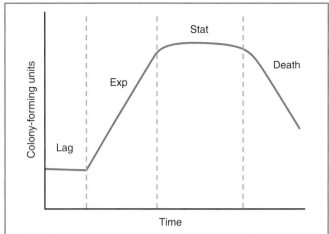

Figure 11-6. Bacterial growth represented by the number of colony-forming units (CFUs) versus time. Growth phases are dependent upon environmental conditions. During the lag phase (Lag), bacteria adapt to growth conditions; individual bacteria are maturing but not yet able to divide. In the exponential phase (Exp), organisms are reproducing at their maximum rate. The growth rate slows during the stationary phase (Stat) owing to depletion of nutrients and exhaustion of available resources. Finally, in the death phase (Death), bacteria run out of nutrients and die.

material takes place, linked to cellular division, so that each daughter cell obtains a full complement of genetic material.

Gene Expression and Regulation

Bacteria lack nuclear membranes, allowing simultaneous transcription of DNA to messenger RNA (mRNA) and translation of proteins. Although bacterial mRNA is short-lived, each message may be translated approximately 20 times prior to degradation by nucleases. mRNA is poly-cistronic, containing genetic information to translate more than one protein. An operon is a group of genes that includes an operator and a common promoter region plus one or more structural genes. Transcriptional regulation occurs through inducer or repressor proteins that interact with structural regions (physical sequences) of the operon to regulate the rate of protein synthesis. Multiple ribosomal units are present on each mRNA, allowing for large numbers of proteins to be produced prior to mRNA destruction. Translation of mRNA usually begins at an AUG start codon preceded by a specific ribosome binding sequence (called the "Shine-Dalgarno region").

KEY POINTS ABOUT BACTERIAL GENETICS

- Bacterial genes are located within the cytoplasm on a super-coiled chromosome as well as on extrachromosomal plasmids.

- Many antibiotic resistance genes are located on plasmids.

- Transfer of genetic material between species may occur through various mechanisms, including conjugation, transduction, and transformation.

- Gene expression and protein synthesis are under tight regulatory control.

●●● BACTERIAL TOXINS: VIRULENCE FACTORS THAT TRIGGER PATHOLOGY

Bacterial toxins are biological virulence factors that prepare the host for colonization. By definition, a toxin triggers a destructive process (Fig. 11-8). Toxins can function in multiple ways, for example, by inhibiting protein synthesis (diphtheria toxin), activating second messenger pathways (*Bacillus anthracis* edema factor or cholera toxin), activating immune responses (*S. aureus* superantigens), damaging cell membranes (*E. coli* hemolysin), or by general action of metalloprotease activity (*Clostridium tetani* tetanus toxin). Toxins come in a variety of forms. LPS is considered a powerful endotoxin; its activity has been attributed to the lipid A portion of the molecule. In contrast to bound endotoxins, bacterial exotoxins are soluble mediators located in the bacterial cytoplasm or periplasm that are either excreted or released during bacterial cell lysis or destruction. A specific class of exotoxins, called

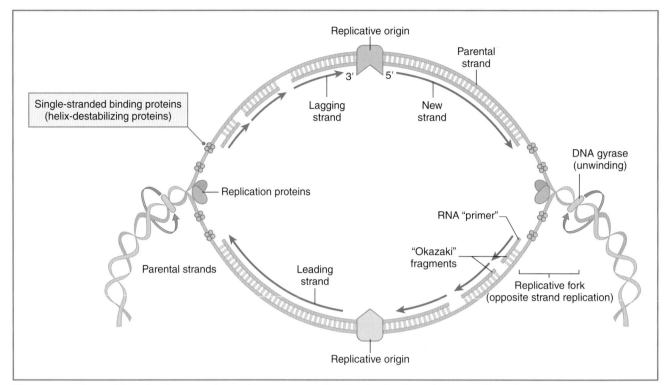

Figure 11-7. Bacterial replication as a three-phase process. Replication begins with unwinding of the DNA beginning at a unique sequence termed the origin of replication. Gyrases (topoisomerases) unwind the chromosome, while single-stranded binding proteins (ssbs) hold open the double helix to allow polymerases to copy the strands through addition of complementary nucleotides in a 5′ to 3′ direction. Bidirectional copying occurs by synthesizing short Okazaki fragments on the lagging strand, which are later connected by specific ligases.

enterotoxins, is toxic to the intestinal tract, causing vomiting and diarrhea. Well-defined toxins (such as enterotoxins, neurotoxins, leukocidins, and hemolysins) are classified in terms of the specific target cell or site affected. Table 11-1 lists major toxins and their mechanism of action.

KEY POINTS ABOUT BACTERIAL TOXINS
- Many bacteria synthesize toxins that serve as primary virulence factors, inducing pathologic damage to host tissue.
- Toxins may function to establish productive colonization conditions and work by damaging host cell membranes, by inhibiting host cell protein synthesis, and by activating secondary messengers that adversely affect host cell function.

●●● MAJOR ANTIMICROBIAL AGENTS AGAINST BACTERIA

Antimicrobial agents can be categorized as molecules that act to kill or inhibit bacterial growth by interfering with (1) cell wall synthesis, (2) ribosomal function and protein synthesis, (3) nucleic acid synthesis, (4) folate synthesis, or (5) plasma membrane integrity. Many useful antimicrobial agents and their mechanisms of action are listed in Table 11-2. Briefly, cell wall synthesis is inhibited by β-lactams, such as penicillins and cephalosporins, which inhibit peptidoglycan polymerization. In addition, vancomycin inhibits synthesis of cell wall substrates. Aminoglycosides, streptomycin, tetracycline, chloramphenicol, erythromycin (clarithromycin, azithromycin), and clindamycin all interfere with ribosome function through binding to the 30S or 50S ribosomal subunit. Quinolones bind to a bacterial complex of DNA and DNA gyrase, blocking DNA replication. Rifampin blocks transcription of mRNA synthesis by binding and inhibiting RNA polymerase. Nitroimidazoles damage DNA. Nalidixic acids (floxacin, ciprofloxacin, norfloxacin) inhibit DNA unwinding needed for DNA synthesis. Sulfonamides and trimethoprim block the synthesis of folate needed for DNA replication. Polymyxins and amphotericin disrupt the plasma membrane, causing leakage. The plasma membrane sterols of fungi are attacked by polyenes (amphotericin) and imidazoles.

Bacterial resistance is a natural outcome of evolution and environmental pressure. Resistance factors can be encoded on plasmids or within the bacterial chromosome. The etiology of antimicrobial resistance may involve mechanisms that limit entry of the drug, changes in the receptor (target) of the drug, or metabolic inactivation of the drug. Bacteria acquire genes conferring antimicrobial resistance in numerous ways including spontaneous DNA mutation, bacterial transformation, and plasmid transfer.

A

B

Figure 11-8. Bacterial toxins function as virulence factors. Two mechanisms for bacterial toxin action include damage to cellular membranes (**A**) and inhibition of protein synthesis (**B**). Damage to cellular membranes, such as by *Staphylococcus aureus* or *Clostridium perfringens* alpha toxin, function by assembling a heptomeric prepore complex on target membranes that undergoes conformational change to disrupt membrane permeability and affect influx and efflux of ions. Inhibition of protein synthesis, as exemplified by *Shigella dysenteriae* Shiga toxin, *Escherichia coli* heat-labile toxin I, and cholera and pertussis toxins, work as substrates for elongation factors and ribosomal RNA.

PHARMACOLOGY

β-Lactam Antibiotics

β-Lactam antibiotics are inhibitors of cell wall synthesis, working to limit transpeptidase and carboxypeptidase action involved in terminal cross-linking of glycopeptides in the formation of the peptidoglycan layer. Penicillins derived from the mold *Penicillium* consist of a β-lactam ring coupled to a thiazolidine ring. Addition of defined side chains to the free amino group produces a range of synthetic antibiotics, including ampicillin and methicillin, which are active against both gram-negative and gram-positive species.

KEY POINTS ABOUT ANTIMICROBIAL AGENTS

- Antimicrobial agents function through inhibition of synthetic pathways required for bacterial growth and via direct damage to bacterial membranes.

- Bacterial antibiotic resistance is a natural phenomenon that may occur by natural mutations to existing genes or through additions to nucleic acid content via transformation or acquisition of plasmid DNA from other bacteria.

TABLE 11-1. Important Bacterial Toxins and Their Mechanism of Action

Toxin	Organism	Mechanism	Clinical Features
Anthrax toxins (edema toxin [EF], lethal toxin [LF])	*Bacillus anthracis*	Adenylyl cyclase (EF), metalloprotease (LF)	Edema and skin necrosis; shock
Adenylate cyclase toxin	*Bordetella pertussis*	Adenylyl cyclase	Tracheobronchitis
Botulinum toxins (C2/C3 toxin)	*Clostridium botulinum*	Blocks release of acetylcholine, ADP-ribosyltransferase	Muscle paralysis, botulism
Toxin A/toxin B	*Clostridium difficile*	Inhibits cytoskeletal action in epithelial cells	Diarrhea, vomiting
Lecithinase (α-toxin; perfringolysin O)	*Clostridium perfringens*	Phospholipase	Gangrene; destruction of phagocytes
Tetanus toxin	*Clostridium tetani*	Blocks release of inhibitory neurotransmitters	Spasms and rigidity of the voluntary muscles; characteristic symptom of "lockjaw"
Diphtheria toxin	*Corynebacterium diphtheriae*	ADP-ribosylates elongation factor-2 (EF-2), inhibiting protein synthesis	Respiratory infection; complicating myocarditis with accompanying neurologic toxicity
CNF-1, CNF-2	*Escherichia coli*	Affects ρ-GTP–binding regulators	Diarrhea
Heat-stable toxin	*Escherichia coli*	Secondary message regulation	Diarrhea
Hemolysin	*Escherichia coli*	Heptameric pore-forming complex (hemolysin)	Urinary tract infections
Shiga-like toxin	*Escherichia coli*	Stops host protein synthesis	Hemolytic uremic syndrome, dysentery
Exotoxin A	*Pseudomonas aeruginosa*	ADP-ribosylates elongation factor-2 (EF-2), inhibiting protein synthesis	Respiratory distress; possible role as virulence factor in lung infections of cystic fibrosis patients
Shiga toxin	*Shigella dysenteriae*	Stops host protein synthesis	Dysentery
α-Toxin	*Staphylococcus aureus*	Heptameric pore-forming complex (hemolysin)	Abscess formation
Toxic shock syndrome toxin 1 (TSST-1)	*Staphylococcus aureus*	Superantigen activates T cell populations, cross-linking V_β TCR and class II MHC	Cytokine cascade elicits shock; capillary leak syndrome and hypotension
Pneumolysin	*Streptococcus pneumoniae*	Pore-forming complex (hemolysin)	Pneumonia
Pyrogenic exotoxin	*Streptococcus pyogenes*	Superantigen activates T cell populations, cross-linking V_β TCR, and class II MHC	Cytokine cascade elicits shock; capillary leak syndrome and hypotension
Streptolysin O	*Streptococcus pyogenes*	Pore-forming complex (hemolysin)	"Strep" throat, scarlet fever
Cholera toxin	*Vibrio cholerae*	Disrupts adenylyl cyclase	Watery diarrhea, loss of electrolytes and fluids

TABLE 11-2. Selected Antimicrobial Agents and General Mechanisms of Action

Cell Wall Synthesis Inhibition	Protein Synthesis Inhibition	Nucleic Acid Function Inhibition	Folic Acid Synthesis Inhibition	Damage to Cell Membrane

Penicillins
  Penicillin G and V
  Ampicillin
  Carbenicillin
  Methicillin
Cephalosporins
Cefamandole
Vancomycin
Bacitracin
Novobiocin
Cycloserine
	Aminoglycosides
	Streptomycin
	  Neomycin
	  Amikacin
	  Kanamycin
	  Gentamicin
	  Tobramycin
	Tetracycline
	  Chlortetracycline
	  Oxytetracycline
	  Doxycycline
	Erythromycin
	  Clarithromycin
	  Azithromycin
	Clindamycin
	Spectinomycin
	Chloramphenicol
	Lincosamides
	Cycloserine
		Quinolones
		Sulfanilamide
		Rifampicin
		Nalidixic acids
		  Floxacin
		  Ciprofloxacin
		  Norfloxacin
		  Levofloxacin
		  Moxifloxacin
		Metronidazole
			Trimethoprim
			Sulfanilamide
			Trimethoprim-sulfamethoxazole
			  (cotrimoxazole)
				Polymyxins
				Amphotericin
				Nystatin
				Imidazole
				Ketoconazole

Clinical Bacteriology

12

CONTENTS

A review of clinically important bacteria includes a wide range of organisms representing pathogens causing disease with complex etiologies. More often than not, the basis of pathogenicity is dependent upon virulence factors produced by the bacteria that mediate environmental conditions and affect host immune function. Opportunistic infections represent organisms that elicit pathogenic responses in immunocompromised or immunosuppressed hosts; in many cases, these bacteria represent normal flora that otherwise rarely cause disease. Table 12-1 outlines the major pathogens of medical significance.

●●● GRAM-POSITIVE COCCI

The *Staphylococcus*, *Streptococcus*, and *Enterococcus* spp are nonmotile, non-spore-forming, gram-positive organisms that cause pyogenic (producing pus) and pyrogenic (producing fever) infections. They represent a major population responsible for cutaneous infections and are causative agents for pathology manifested as systemic disease. Typical skin lesions associated with pyogenic gram-positive organisms include abscesses with central necrosis and pus formation. These include boils, furuncles, and impetigo (cutaneous, pustular eruptions), carbuncles (subcutaneous) and erysipelas (deep-red, diffuse inflammation), paronychias (nailbed infection), and styes (eyelid infection). Systemic infections include bacteremia, food poisoning, endocarditis, toxic shock syndrome, arthritis, and osteomyelitis. The pathogenic mechanisms for clinical disease occur through a combination of toxins and enzymes produced by organisms and relative effects on immune cells involved in combating localized infections. For example, staphylococci produce multiple virulence factors, including exotoxins that regulate cytokines, leukocidins that kill polymorphonuclear cells, and α-toxins (hemolysins) that contribute to local tissue destruction and lysing of red blood cells (Fig. 12-1).

TABLE 12-1. Major Bacterial Pathogens of Medical Interest

Bacterial Type	Description	Example
Gram-positive coccus	Fermentative	
	Catalase-positive	*Staphylococcus*
	Catalase-negative	*Streptococcus*
		Enterococcus
	Oxidative	*Micrococcus*
Gram-negative coccus	Aerobic, non-spore-forming	*N. gonorrhoeae, N. meningitidis, Veillonella*
Gram-positive rod	Endospore-forming	*Bacillus*
		Clostridium
	Regular, non-endospore-forming	*Lactobacillus*
		Listeria
		Erysipelothrix
	Irregular, non-endospore-forming	*Corynebacterium*
Aerobic Gram-negative rod	Enterobacteriaceae	*E. coli*
		Shigella
		Salmonella
		Yersinia
		Edwardsiella
		Citrobacter
		Klebsiella
		Enterobacter
		Serratia
		Proteus
		Morganella
		Providencia
	Respiratory tract	*H. influenzae*
		L. pneumophila
		B. pertussis
	Zoonotic origin	*P. multocida*
		Brucella spp
		F. tularensis
	Nonfermentative	*Pseudomonas*
		Acinetobacter
	Miscellaneous gram-negative rods	*V. cholerae*
		C. jejuni
		H. pylori
Anaerobic Gram-negative rods	Digestive tract	*Bacteroides*
	Pleuropulmonary	*Fusobacterium*
Spirochetes	Spirochaetaceae	*Treponema* (syphilis)
		Borrelia (Lyme disease)
		B. recurrentis, B. hermsii (relapsing fever, antigenic change)
Obligate intracellular pathogen	Atypical cell wall	*Chlamydia*
		Rickettsia
		Ehrlichia
		Coxiella
Acid-fast organism	Mycolic acid cell wall	*M. tuberculosis, M. avium, M. leprae*
	No mycolic acids in cell wall	*Nocardia*
	Intestinal Coccidia	*Cryptosporidium, Cyclospora, Isospora*
Other pathogens	No cell wall	*Mycoplasma*

Staphylococci

The staphylococci are facultative anaerobes, morphologically occurring in grape-like clusters. They are major components of the normal flora of skin and nose and are catalase-positive. *Staphylococcus aureus* (coagulase-positive) is one of the most common causes of opportunistic infections in the hospital and community, including pneumonia, osteomyelitis, septic arthritis, bacteremia, endocarditis, and skin infections. In addition, ingested food contaminated with *S. aureus* enterotoxin can readily lead to vomiting, nausea, diarrhea, and abdominal pain. *S. aureus* produces TSST-1, a super-

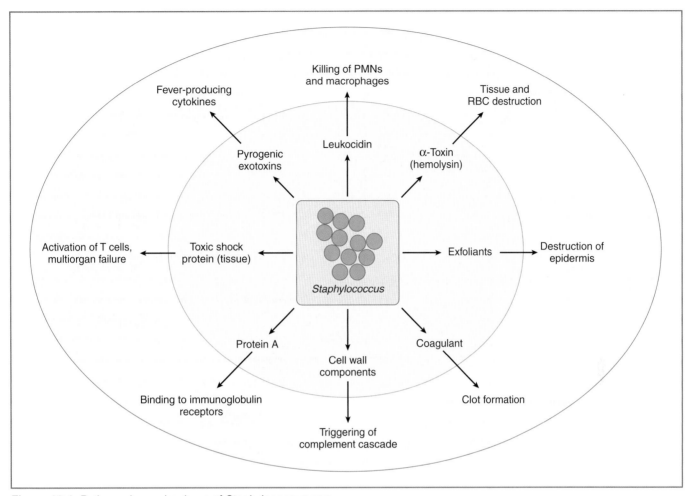

Figure 12-1. Pathogenic mechanisms of *Staphylococcus* spp.

antigen that has been directly linked to toxic shock syndrome. It also produces an exfoliative toxin that causes scalded skin syndrome in babies. *S. aureus* produces various exotoxins as well as tissue-degrading enzymes involved in disease spreading (lipase and hyaluronidase), and protein A, which binds to the Fc portion of IgG, thus inhibiting induction of phagocytosis by PMNs and macrophages and induction of complement cascades.

Staphylococcus epidermidis is a less common cause of opportunistic infection than *S. aureus* and is relevant as a mediator of nosocomial infections. *S. epidermidis* is also a major component of the skin flora and mucous membranes, can easily be cultured from wounds and blood, and is commonly found on catheter tips. A closely related staphylococcal species, *S. saprophyticus*, is a major cause of urinary tract infections in young women. Both *S. epidermidis* and *S. saprophyticus* are coagulase-negative.

Streptococci and Enterococci

The *Streptococcus* spp are subdivided into four groups with *overlapping* ability to cause clinical disease ranging from pharyngitis and general cellulitis to toxic shock syndrome and severe sepsis. The streptococci of medical importance may be identified according to their hemolytic patterns or

according to antigenic differences in carbohydrates located within their cell wall. All streptococci are catalase-negative and exhibit hemolysins of type α or β (streptolysin O and streptolysin S). Group A streptococci (*Streptococcus pyogenes*) is the most clinically important member of the *Streptococcus* spp; *S. pyogenes* is the causative agent of pharyngeal infection, acute rheumatic fever (nonsuppurative disease of the heart and joints), and glomerulonephritis. In addition, it is the etiologic agent of scarlet fever, with erythrogenic (pyrogenic) toxins causing characteristic rash. One of the pyrogenic toxins is a superantigen, causing mitogenic T-cell response in a non-antigen-specific mediated manner. Other toxins (pyrogenic toxins A, B, and C) when released result in severe edema and necrotizing myositis and fasciitis. Some of the pathogenic mechanisms are depicted in Figure 12-2.

Streptococcus agalactiae (group B streptococcus) readily colonizes the vaginal region and is a common cause of neonatal bacteremia and sepsis, pneumonia, and meningitis due to transmission from mother to child before or after childbirth. The group D streptococci include *Streptococcus bovis* and the enterococci. *Enterococcus faecalis* (previously identified as *Streptococcus faecalis*) is a causative agent of urinary and biliary tract infections and also contributes to bacteremia and endocarditis. *Enterococcus faecalis* is

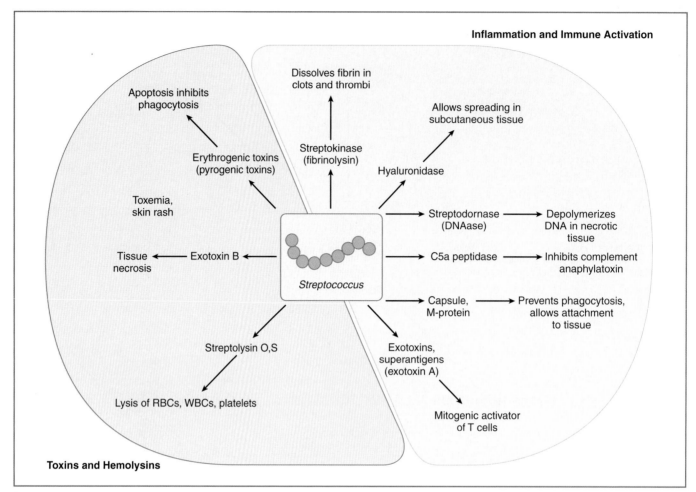

Figure 12-2. Pathogenic mechanisms for group A streptococci (*Streptococcus pyogenes*).

γ-hemolytic and has been linked to colon carcinomas. The bacterium *Streptococcus viridans* is responsible for approximately half of all cases of bacterial endocarditis. Members of this group include *Streptococcus mutans*, *Streptococcus sanguis*, and *Streptococcus salivarius*. Although these organisms are normally found as oral bacterial flora, entry into the bloodstream can lead to fever and embolic events. Group C streptococcus (*Streptococcus equisimilis*, *Streptococcus zooepidemicus*, *Streptococcus equi*, *Streptococcus dysgalactiae*) primarily causes diseases of animals and poses little threat to immunocompetent hosts. Likewise, groups E, F, G, H, and K-U spp rarely cause pathogenic disease.

Streptococcus pneumoniae (referred to as pneumococci) is a leading cause of pneumonia, often with onset after damage to the upper respiratory tract (e.g., following viral infection). Although *S. pneumoniae* is hemolytic, there is no group antigen and no main exotoxins that contribute to pathogenesis. The organism often spreads, causing bacteremia and meningitis, and may also cause middle ear infections (otitis media). *S. pneumoniae* has an antiphagocytic capsule (antigenically effective as a vaccine target) and produces a pneumolysin that degrades red blood cells to allow productive spread from respiratory membranes to the blood. It also produces an IgA protease, which more readily allows colonization of respiratory mucosa. Complement activation by teichoic acid may explain the attraction of large numbers of inflammatory cells to the focal site of infection.

Other Gram-Positive Cocci of Medical Importance

The *Micrococcus* spp include organisms that may produce pathology in immunocompromised individuals (those with neutropenia, SCID, or acquired immunodeficiency). Of these, *Stomatococcus mucilaginosus*, normally a soil-residing organism, may induce disease. *Peptostreptococcus* is an anaerobic counterpart of *Streptococcus*. Peptostreptococci are small bacteria that grow in chains, usually are nonpathogenic, and are found as normal flora of the skin, urethra, and urogenital tract. Under opportunistic conditions, they can infect bones, joints, and soft tissue. *Peptostreptococcus magnus* is the species most often isolated from infected tissues.

●●● GRAM-NEGATIVE COCCI
Neisseria

The *Neisseria* genus consists of aerobic, non-spore-forming gram-negative diplococcobacilli that reside in mucous membranes. They are nonmotile, oxidase-positive, glucose-fermenting microbes that require a moist environment and warm temperatures to achieve optimum growth. The two most clinically significant members of the genus *Neisseria* are *Neisseria gonorrhoeae* (gonococcus) and *Neisseria meningitidis* (meningococcus). Infection by *N. gonorrhoeae* is referred to as a gonococcal infection, transmitted by intimate contact with the mucous membrane. In infected males, the disease is characterized by urethritis with a urethral pus discharge; if left untreated, resulting complications such as prostatitis and periurethral abscess may occur. Females with gonorrhea exhibit vaginal discharge (cervicitis or vulvovaginitis) with accompanying abdominal pain and nonmenstrual bleeding. As with most other sexually transmitted diseases, gonorrhea is prevalent in young adult and homosexual populations. *N. gonorrhoeae* is sensitive to antibiotics; the common association with chlamydial infection dictates employing a therapeutic regimen of cephalosporin (ceftriaxone) and a tetracycline or quinolone to kill organisms. If left untreated, *N. gonorrhoeae* can cause meningitis with septicemia, and resulting arthritis and acute endocarditis upon further dissemination of organisms.

N. meningitidis colonizes the nasopharynx and is the second most prevalent causative agent of meningitis in the United States. Upon invasion of blood, it may cause purpura, endotoxic shock, and meningitis with characteristic inflammation of membranes covering the central nervous system (CNS). Early symptoms are headache, fever, and vomiting; death can quickly follow owing to focal cerebral involvement from the highly toxic lipopolysaccharide. *N. meningitidis* also has an antiphagocytic capsule, which contributes to its virulence. Different strains of *N. meningitidis* are classified by their capsular polysaccharides, with nine divisible serogroups (A, B, C, D, X, Y, Z, W135, and 29E). *N. meningitidis*, as well as *N. gonorrhoeae*, produces IgA proteases that also promote virulence. Organisms can assume a carrier status with the disease actually developing in very few carriers. Most infected patients can be treated with penicillin G, while rifampin may be used prophylactically to prevent reactivation of disease.

Veillonella

Veillonella spp are nonmotile, gram-negative diplococci that are the anaerobic counterpart of *Neisseria*. *Veillonella* is part of the normal flora of the mouth and gastrointestinal tract and may be found in the vagina as well. Although of limited pathogenicity, *Veillonella* is often mistaken for the more serious gonococcal infection. *Veillonella* spp are often regarded as contaminants; they are often associated with oral infections; bite wounds; head, neck, and various soft tissue infections; and they have also been implicated as pathogens in infections of the sinuses, lungs, heart, bone, and CNS. Recent reports have also indicated their isolation in pure culture in septic arthritis and meningitis.

●●● AEROBIC GRAM-POSITIVE BACILLI

Bacillus

Bacillus is a genus of gram-positive bacteria that are ever-present in soil, water, and airborne dust. *Bacillus* may be found as a natural flora in the intestines. *Bacillus* has the ability to produce endospores under stressful environmental conditions. The organism is nonmotile and nonhemolytic and is highly pathogenic. The only other known spore-producing bacterium is *Clostridium*. Although most species of *Bacillus* are harmless saprophytes, two species are considered medically significant; *Bacillus anthracis* and *Bacillus cereus*. *B. anthracis* is a nonhemolytic, nonmotile, catalase-positive bacterium that causes anthrax in cows, sheep, and sometimes humans. Under the microscope, *B. anthracis* cells appear to have square ends and seem to be attached by a joint to other cells. Anthrax is transmitted to humans by cutaneous contact (infection of abrasions) with endospores, or more rarely by inhalation. Rare cases of gastrointestinal infection may occur. Cutaneous anthrax causes ulceration, with a distinctive black necrotic center surrounded by an edematous areola with pustules. Pulmonary and gastrointestinal infections are more likely to result in toxemia. *B. anthracis* secretes three toxins to help evade host immune response through exertion of apoptotic effect on responding cells (Fig. 12-3). Two of these toxins are edema factor (EF) and lethal factor (LF), both of which have negative effects via enzymatic modification of substrates within the cytosol of the host cell. Protective factor (PA), the third component, binds to a cellular receptor, termed anthrax toxin receptor (ATR), and functions in transporting both EF and LF into host cells.

Unlike *B. anthracis*, *B. cereus* is a motile, catalase-positive bacterium that is the causative agent of a toxin-mediated food poisoning. It is a common soil and water saprophyte that, upon ingestion, releases two toxins into the gastrointestinal tract that cause vomiting and diarrhea; the clinical manifestations are similar to those of *Staphylococcus* food poisoning. One of the endotoxins is similar to the heat-labile toxin of *Escherichia coli*, with associated activation of cAMP-dependent protein kinase activity in enterocytes underlying watery diarrhea production. Proper cold storage of food is recommended immediately after preparation to limit growth and toxin production.

Lactobacillus

Lactobacillus is a gram-positive, facultatively anaerobic, nonmotile, non-spore-forming bacterium that ferments

---

PATHOLOGY

Pus and Abscess Formation

An accumulation of pus in an enclosed tissue space is known as an abscess. Pus, a whitish-yellow substance is found in regions of bacterial infection including superficial infections such as pimples. Pus consists of macrophages and neutrophils, bacterial debris, dead and dying cell and necrotic tissue. Necrosis is caused by released lysosomes, including lipases, carbohydrases, proteases, and nucleases.

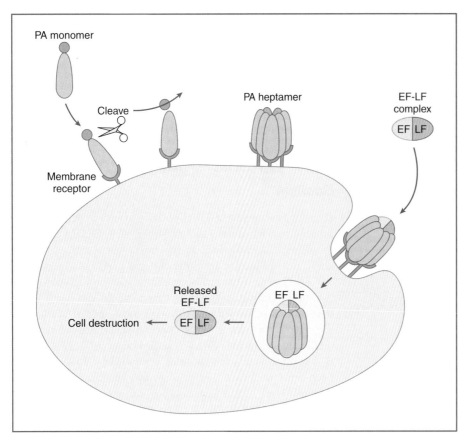

Figure 12-3. Mechanisms of anthrax toxin. Assembly of lethal *Bacillus anthracis* toxin on the cell surface causes anthrax poisoning. The bacteria produce three proteins which, when combined, kill cells. The proteins—protective antigen (PA; monomers forming a heptamer prepore), lethal factor (LF; primary protease-cleaving mitogen-activated protein kinase) and edema factor (EF; adenylate cyclase, converting ATP into cAMP)—are not toxic as monomers released by the bacteria, but they cause cell disruption upon interacting.

PATHOLOGY

Pathophysiology of Diarrhea

The causes of diarrhea may be identified as defects in absorption, secretion, or motility. Factors that alter the normal transit of a meal through the alimentary canal affect the consistency of the fecal contents; increases in motility are correlated with diarrhea. Infection that alters the function of the enterocytes of the small intestine leads to massive water flux to the colon. Specific effectors that increase cAMP levels in enterocytes stimulate secretion of chloride and bicarbonate, with associated sodium and water secretion.

glucose into lactose, earning its name. The most common application of *Lactobacillus* is for dairy production. This genus contains several species that belong to the natural flora of the vagina, with other related organisms found in the colon and mouth. *Lactobacillus* derives lactic acid from glucose, creating an acidic environment that inhibits growth of other bacterial species, which contributes to urogenital infections. In the mouth, colonization may affect dentition; if the caries infection in enamel goes unchecked, acid dissolution can advance cavitation extending through the dentin (the component of the tooth located under the enamel) to the pulp tissue, which is rich in nerves and blood vessels. In rare cases of infection, treatment usually consists of high doses of penicillin in combination with gentamicin.

Listeria

Listeria is a gram-positive, catalase-positive rod (diphtheroid) that is not capable of forming endospores. Two species are of human pathogenic significance: *Listeria monocytogenes* and *Listeria ivanovii*. In particular, *L. monocytogenes* causes meningitis and sepsis in newborns and accounts for 10% of community-acquired bacterial meningitis in adults. *Listeria* is also the cause of diarrheogenic disease in humans, with those infected suffering from vomiting, nausea, and diarrhea. Ingestion of *Listeria* from unpasteurized milk products can lead to bacteremia and septicemia with meningoencephalitis. When transmitted across the placenta to the fetus, infection can lead to placentitis, neonatal septicemia, and possible abortion. At-risk individuals for listeriosis include newborns, pregnant women and their fetuses, the elderly, and persons lacking a healthy immune system. The bacterium usually causes septicemia and meningitis in patients with suppressed immune function. Antibiotics are recommended for treatment of infection because most strains of *Listeria* are sensitive to ampicillin plus an aminoglycoside. Identification utilizes β-hemolysis on blood agar plates.

Erysipelothrix

Erysipelothrix rhusiopathiae is a common veterinary pathogen; however, infection of human hosts occurs. In humans, *Erysipelothrix* is an aerobic, non-spore-forming, gram-positive bacillus that has been linked to skin infections in meat and fish handlers; the most common presentation is cellulitis (erysipeloid), a localized cutaneous infection. A more serious condition may occur involving lesions that progress from the initial site of infection or appear in remote areas. A severe form of disease is a septicemia that is almost always linked to endocarditis. Treatment usually consists of penicillin G, ampicillin, cephalothin, or other β-lactam antibiotics. Most clinical strains are resistant to vancomycin.

Corynebacteria

The coryneform group includes several genera of non-spore-forming rods that are ubiquitous in nature. They are gram-positive bacteria that include the clinically important *Actinomyces* and *Corynebacterium*. *Corynebacterium* spp are nonmotile, facultatively anaerobic bacteria that are usually saprophytic and cause little harm to humans. However, the *Corynebacterium diphtheriae* can be pathogenic, producing the toxin that causes diphtheria, a disease of the upper respiratory system. Although other species of *Corynebacterium* can inhabit the mucous membrane, *C. diphtheria* is unique in its exotoxin formation. Pathogenesis manifests as inflammatory exudates that may spread infection to the postnasal cavity or the larynx and cause respiratory obstruction. Bacilli do not penetrate deeply into underlying tissues; rather, a powerful exotoxin is produced that has a special affinity for heart, muscle, nerve endings, and the adrenal glands. The diphtheria toxin is a heat-stable polypeptide composed of two fragments, which together inhibit polypeptide chain elongation at the ribosome. Inhibition of protein synthesis is probably responsible for both necrotic and neurotoxic effects. Patients have malaise, fatigue, fever, and sore throat; infection manifesting as anterior nasal diphtheria presents with a thick nasal discharge. *C. diphtheriae* is sensitive to penicillin, tetracycline, rifampicin, and clindamycin. The bacteria may be viewed microscopically using Löffler's methylene blue stain. An antitoxin should be administered at the first evidence of infection and should not await laboratory confirmation.

Other medically important coryneforms include *Corynebacterium ulcerans* and *Arcanobacterium haemolyticum*, causative agents of acute pharyngeal infections; *Corynebacterium pseudotuberculosis*, involved in subacute lymphadenitis; *Corynebacterium minutissimum*, associated with infections of the stratum corneum, leading to erythrasma (scaly red patches); and *Corynebacterium jeikeium*, which has been implicated in endocarditis, neutropenia, and hematologic malignancy.

●●● ANAEROBIC GRAM-POSITIVE BACILLI

Clostridium

Clostridium spp are gram-positive, anaerobic spore-forming rods that are motile in their vegetative form. They are ubiquitous in soil. Physically, they appear as long thick rods with a bulge at one end. *Clostridium* grows well at body temperature; under stressed environments the bacteria produce spores that tolerate extreme conditions. These bacteria secrete powerful exotoxins responsible for diseases including those causing tetanus, botulism, and gas gangrene. The four clinically important species are *Clostridium tetani*, *Clostridium botulinum*, *Clostridium perfringens*, and *Clostridium difficile*.

C. tetani causes tetanus (lockjaw) in humans. *C. tetani* spores will germinate in an anaerobic environment to form active *C. tetani* cells with a drumstick-shaped appearance. Growth in dead tissue allows production and release of an exotoxin (tetanospasmin) that causes nervous system irregularities interfering with spinal cord synaptic reflexes. The toxin blocks inhibitory mechanisms that regulate muscle contraction, leading to constant skeletal muscle contraction. Prolonged infection leads to eventual respiratory failure with high mortality if left untreated. Immunization is highly effective in preventing *C. tetani* infections in both children and adults.

C. botulinum produces one of the most potent neurotoxins and is the cause of deadly botulism food poisoning. Airborne *Clostridium* spores can find their way into foods that will be placed in anaerobic storage. Immediate symptoms of infection include muscular weakness with blurred vision, developing into an afebrile neurologic disorder with characteristic descending paralysis due to blocked release of acetylcholine (Fig. 12-4). Immediate treatment with antitoxin is required. Infantile botulism is much milder than the adult version; honey is a common source of spores that can germinate in the intestinal tract of children.

C. perfringens is a nonmotile, invasive pathogen responsible for gas gangrene (clostridial myositis or myonecrosis). The organism is commonly found among the gastrointestinal tract flora and can be found colonizing the skin, especially in the perirectal region. The organism can easily invade wounds that come into contact with soil. *C. perfringens* cells proliferate after spore germination occurs, releasing a variety of virulence factors that can degrade tissue. *C. perfringens* produces a lecithinase capable of lysing cells, a protease, hyaluronidase, collagenase, and other hemolysins. The combination of virulence factors produced is strain dependent. All strains produce lecithinase (also called α-toxin), which plays a central role in pathogenesis of gas gangrene. Lecithinase can lyse white blood cells, enhancing its ability to evade the immune system and spread through tissues. Released exotoxin causes necrosis of the surrounding tissue. The boxcar shaped bacteria themselves produce gas, which leads to a bubbly deformation of infected tissues. Treatment of histotoxic *C. perfringens* consists of penicillin G (to kill the organism), hyperbaric O_2, administration of antitoxin, and débridement of infected areas.

C. difficile is a motile, obligate, anaerobic or microaerophilic, gram-positive, spore-forming, rod-shaped bacillus. *C. difficile*–associated disease occurs when the normal intestinal flora is altered, allowing the bacteria to flourish in the intestinal tract and produce a toxin that causes a watery diarrhea.

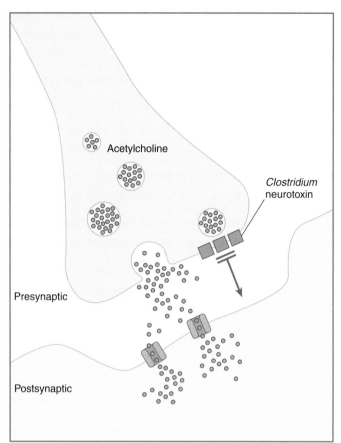

Figure 12-4. Action of clostridial neurotoxins. *Clostridium* produces an endopeptidase that blocks the release of acetylcholine at the myoneural junction. Muscle paralysis is the result. Both the botulinum toxin and the tetanus toxin interfere with vesicle formation at synaptic junctions, resulting in muscle spasms and loss of neural signal.

C. difficile is recognized as a chief cause of nosocomial (hospital-acquired) diarrhea. Infections can appear through the use of broad-spectrum antibiotics, which lower the relative amount of other normal gut flora, thereby allowing *C. difficile* proliferation and infection into the large intestine. The bacterium then releases two enterotoxins (colitis toxins A and B) that are cytotoxic to enterocytes, thus causing a pseudomembranous colitis by destroying the intestinal lining. The end result is diarrhea. The preferred method of treatment is oral vancomycin or metronidazole plus rehydration.

Actinomyces

Actinomyces spp are gram-positive, obligate anaerobes known to reside in the mouth and intestinal tract. They are morphologically similar to fungus in that they form filamentous branches. Pathology due to proliferation of organisms usually occurs following injury or trauma to tissue, resulting in actinomycosis (abscess formation and swelling at the site of infection). Microscopic examination of pus will reveal exudates with granular texture caused by sulfur granules, resulting from the bacterium and its waste. *Actinomyces israelii* is most commonly associated with actino-

mycosis; however, other *Actinomyces* bacteria are capable of causing disease. Actinomycosis can be treated with penicillin.

Bifidobacterium

Bifidobacteria are anaerobic, gram-positive bacilli rarely associated with infection. *Bifidobacterium dentium*, a normal inhabitant of the gut flora, is the only pathogenic species reported. Microscopically, these organisms appear bone shaped, making them easy to identify. They are obligate anaerobes and require very low O_2 tension to survive and achieve moderate growth.

Eubacterium and *Propionibacterium*

Eubacterium spp are of only minor clinical importance. They are normal flora of the intestinal tract and cause infection under opportunistic conditions. *Eubacterium lentum* is the species that is most often isolated, and it has been linked to endocarditis. Biochemical testing can distinguish *Eubacterium* from the other gram-positive, anaerobic rods. *Propionibacterium* spp are common gram-positive anaerobes isolated in the laboratory. *Propionibacterium acnes* is typically noninvasive and harmless, but it has pathogenic potential and has been linked to endocarditis, wound infections, and abscesses. Despite its name, *P. acnes* is not the causative agent of acne, although it may infect acne sites. Microscopically, *Propionibacterium* clumps together and shows a minor branching tendency, with uneven gram-staining patterns. Colonies grow best in anaerobic or microaerophilic environments on blood agar.

●●● AEROBIC GRAM-NEGATIVE BACILLI

Enterobacteriaceae

Members of the Enterobacteriaceae family are among the most pathogenic and commonly encountered organisms in clinical microbiology. They are large, gram-negative rods usually associated with intestinal infections, typically, meningitis, bacillary dysentery, typhoid, and food poisoning. They are oxidase-negative, and all members of this family are glucose fermenters and nitrate reducers. The pathogenicity of each enteric member may be determined by its ability to metabolize lactose. The various genera of the Enterobacteriaceae family most commonly encountered in the clinical laboratory are presented here.

HISTOLOGY

Histology of the Intestine

The intestine is histologically characterized by the presence of the muscularis propria with Auerbach's plexus between the inner circular and outer longitudinal smooth muscle layers. Meissner's plexus is similar in function but found in submucosal areas.

Escherichia coli

E. coli is the main cause of human urinary tract infections (UTIs), and it has been linked to sepsis, pneumonia, meningitis, and traveler's diarrhea. It is part of the normal flora of the intestinal tract; *E. coli* produces vitamin K in the large intestine, which plays a crucial role in food digestion. Pathogenic strains of *E. coli* have a powerful cell wall–associated endotoxin that causes septic shock, and two enterotoxins. One enterotoxin is a heat-labile (LT) molecule that stimulates ADP-ribosylation via adenylate cyclase activity, leading to dysregulation of chloride ions in the gut. A heat-stable toxin (ST) also contributes to diarrheal illness. Treatment of *E. coli* infections with antibiotics sometimes leads to release of additional factors causing severe shock, which is potentially fatal. At the species level, *E. coli* and *Shigella* are indistinguishable, with much overlap between diseases caused by the two organisms.

Four etiologically distinct diseases are defined according to clinical symptoms. Enteropathogenic *E. coli* (EPEC) is commonly found associated with infant diarrhea due to destruction of microvilli without invasion of the organism, leading to fever, diarrhea, vomiting, and nausea, usually with nonbloody stools. Enterotoxigenic *E. coli* (ETEC) is the cause of traveler's diarrhea due to the plasmid-encoded LT and ST toxins. Enteroinvasive *E. coli* (EIEC) produces a dysentery indistinguishable clinically from shigellosis. Enterohemorrhagic *E. coli* (EHEC), usually of serotype O157:H7, produces a hemorrhagic colitis characterized by bloody and copious diarrhea with few leukocytes in afebrile patients.

Shigella

Shigella spp are closely related to *Escherichia*. *Shigella* usually is distinguishable from *E. coli*, since it is anaerogenic (does not produce gas from carbohydrates) and lactose-negative. *Shigella* is an invasive, facultative, gram-negative rod pathogen; four species may be designated based on serologic identity, all of which cause bloody diarrhea accompanied by fever and intestinal pain. The members of the species causing shigellosis are *Shigella dysenteriae* (serotype A), *Shigella flexneri* (serotype B), *Shigella boydii* (serotype C), and *Shigella sonnei* (serotype D). Serotype D is primarily responsible for shigellosis. Following infection, dysentery results from bacteria damaging epithelial layers lining the intestine, with release of mucus and blood and attraction of leukocytes. A neurotoxic, enterotoxic, cytotoxic, chromosome-encoded Shiga toxin is responsible for the pathology. The toxin inhibits protein synthesis. Managing dehydration is of primary concern. Indeed, mild diarrhea often is not recognized as shigellosis. Patients with severe dysentery are usually treated with antibiotics (e.g., ampicillin).

Salmonella

Salmonella spp are facultative, gram-negative, non-lactose-fermenting rods. Transmission of *Salmonella* bacteria occurs through eating of uncooked meats and eggs, with chickens serving as a major reservoir in the food chain. Ingestion of contaminated foods can cause intestinal infection leading to diarrhea, vomiting, and chills. *Salmonella* spp are classified according to their surface antigens. In the United States, *Salmonella typhimurium* (gastroenteritis) and *Salmonella enteritidis* (enterocolitis) are the two leading causes of salmonellosis (inflammation of the intestine caused by *Salmonella*). *S. typhi* causes typhoid fever (enteric fever), which is characterized by fever, diarrhea, and inflammation of infected organs. Most *Salmonella* infections can be treated with ciprofloxacin or ceftriaxone.

Yersinia

Yersinia is an invasive pathogen that can infiltrate the intestinal lining to enter the lymphatic system and the blood supply. Infection through ingestion of contaminated foods causes severe intestinal inflammation (yersiniosis). *Yersinia enterocolitica* is a urease-positive organism associated with diarrhea, fever, and abdominal pain (gastroenteritis) caused by release of its enterotoxin. A similar but less severe disease is caused by *Yersinia pseudotuberculosis*. *Y. pseudotuberculosis* (formerly called *Pasteurella pseudotuberculosis*) is pathogenic, causing mesenteric lymphadenitis in humans. Antibiotic treatment consists of aminoglycosides, chloramphenicol, or tetracycline.

Although not a true enteric pathogen, *Yersinia pestis* is included as a historical note as the causative agent for the bubonic, pneumonic, and septicemic plagues. Human contraction of *bubonic plague* may occur via flea bites, with transfer of disease from a rodent reservoir. *Y. pestis* is a urease-negative organism that has cell wall protein-lipoprotein complexes (V and W antigens) that inhibit phagocytosis, and it releases a toxin during infection that inhibits electron transport chain function. Swelling of the lymph nodes and delirium are observed within a few days of infection, followed by pneumonia characterized by high fever, cough with bloody sputum, chills, and severe chest pains. Death will occur if it is left untreated. Effective antibiotic treatment consists of streptomycin and gentamicin.

Other Pathogenic Enterobacteriaceae

Edwardsiella spp are biochemically similar to *E. coli*; however, *Edwardsiella tarda* has the distinction of producing hydrogen sulfide (H_2S); it can cause gastroenteritis and infect open wounds in humans. *Citrobacter* is part of the normal gut flora; *Citrobacter freundii* can cause diarrhea and possibly extraintestinal infections. *Citrobacter diversus* may cause meningitis in newborns. *Klebsiella* spp are large, nonmotile bacteria that produce a heat-stable enterotoxin. *Klebsiella pneumoniae* causes pneumonia with characteristic bloody sputum, and urinary tract infections in catheterized patients. *Enterobacter* includes multiple species of highly motile bacteria that normally reside in the intestinal tract. They are biochemically similar to *Klebsiella* and can cause opportunistic infections of the urinary tract. *Enterobacter aerogenes* and *Enterobacter cloacae* are two examples of pathogens that are associated with urinary tract and respiratory tract infections. Members of the *Serratia* genus produce pathogenic enzymes including DNase, lipase, and gelatinase.

Serratia marcescens causes urinary tract infections, wound infections, and pneumonia. *Proteus* spp are highly motile and form irregular "swarming" colonies. *Proteus mirabilis* and *Proteus vulgaris* cause wound and urinary tract infections, especially important in the immunocompromised or immunosuppressed host. Of the *Morganella* spp, *Morganella morganii* is clinically important and can cause urinary tract and wound infections as well as diarrhea. Finally, *Providencia* spp have been associated with nosocomial (hospital-acquired) urinary tract infections; *Providencia alcalifaciens* has been associated with diarrhea in children.

Haemophilus

Respiratory tract infections caused by pleomorphic, aerobic, gram-negative rods include organisms of the *Haemophilus*, *Legionella*, and *Bordetella* spp. The *Haemophilus* genus represents a group of gram-negative rods that grow on blood agar, requiring blood factors X (an iron-tetrapyrrole such as hemin) and V (NAD+ or NADP+). Morphologically, *Haemophilus* bacteria usually appear as tiny coccobacilli, designated as pleomorphic bacteria because of their multiple morphologies. *Haemophilus* spp are classified by their capsule into six different serologic groups (a to f). Infection by *Haemophilus influenzae* is common in children and causes secondary respiratory infections in individuals who already have the flu. *H. influenzae* may present with or without a pathogenic polysaccharide capsule and is present as normal flora residing in the nose and pharynx. Strains without a capsule usually cause mild, contained infections (otitis media, sinusitis); however, type b encapsulated *H. influenzae* can cause meningitis with fever, headache, and stiff neck. Other presentations occur as cellulitis, arthritis, or sepsis. Prior to the introduction of a highly effective vaccine, *H. influenzae* was the most common cause of bacterial meningitis in children under the age of 5 years in developed countries (*S. pneumoniae* and *N. meningitides* now are more important). In less well developed countries, *H. influenzae* infection is still a major problem. Respiratory infection may spread from the blood to eventually infect CNS tissue. *Haemophilus* infection is typically associated with other lung disorders (chronic bronchitis, pneumonia) as well as with bacteremia and conjunctivitis. Cephalosporins are used in treatment. Other species of clinical interest are *Haemophilus aegyptius*, which cause pinkeye (conjunctivitis), and *Haemophilus ducreyi*, which causes a sexually transmitted disease characterized by painful genital ulcers (chancroid).

Legionella

The genus *Legionella* was headlined in the mid-1970s when an outbreak of pneumonia at an American Legion convention led to multiple deaths (legionnaires' disease). The causative agent, *Legionella pneumophila*, is a gram-negative intracellular bacterium that produces off-white, circular colonies. Respiratory transmission leads to infection characterized by the gradual onset of fever, chills, and a dry cough; eventual progression to severe pneumonia may occur, with possible spread to the gastrointestinal tract and CNS. Advanced infections are characterized by diarrhea, nausea, disorientation, and confusion. *L. pneumophila* is associated with Pontiac fever, evidenced by generally mild flu-like symptoms that do not develop and spread beyond the lungs. *L. pneumophila* infections are easily treated with erythromycin. *Legionella micdadei* is similar to *L. pneumophila* but does not produce β-lactamase. *L. micdadei* causes similar flu-like symptoms and pneumonia.

Bordetella

Bordetella organisms are small, gram-negative coccobacilli. They are strict aerobes. The most clinically important species is *Bordetella pertussis*, which causes whooping cough. The organism enters the respiratory tract after inhalation and destroys the ciliated epithelial cells of the trachea and bronchi through various toxins. These toxins include the pertussis toxin (exotoxin) that activates host cell production of cAMP to modulate cell protein synthesis regulation, a tracheal cytotoxin that causes destruction of ciliated epithelial cells, and a cell surface hemagglutinin to assist in bacterial binding to the host cells. Antimicrobial therapy for whooping cough usually consists of erythromycin.

Two other species of *Bordetella* of clinical importance are *Bordetella parapertussis*, a respiratory pathogen that causes mild pharyngitis, and *Bordetella bronchiseptica*, which causes pneumonia and otitis media.

●●● ORGANISMS OF ZOONOTIC ORIGIN

Pasteurella

Infection of the lungs with *Pasteurella* spp, usually *Pasteurella multocida* or *Pasteurella haemolytica*, causes pneumonic pasteurellosis, a fulminating, fatal lobar pneumonia. Other pathologies attributed to these organisms include septicemic pasteurellosis and a hemorrhagic septicemia. *P. multocida* is a member of the genus of gram-negative, facultatively anaerobic, ovoid to rod-shaped bacteria of the family Pasteurellaceae. It is an extracellular parasite that may be cultured on chocolate agar and typically produces a foul odor. *P. multocida* commonly infects humans and is acquired usually through scratches or bites from cat or dogs. Patients tend to exhibit swelling, cellulitis, and some bloody drainage at the wound site, as well as abscesses and septicemias. Infection in nearby joints can cause swelling and arthritis. *P. haemolytica*, a species that is part of the normal flora of cattle and sheep, is the etiologic agent of hemorrhagic septicemia. Both *P. multocida* and *P. haemolytica* are susceptible to penicillin, tetracycline, and chloramphenicol.

Brucella

Brucella is an aerobic, gram-negative coccobacillus that is the causative agent of brucellosis. Four species infect humans:

Brucella abortus (cattle), *Brucella suis* (swine), *Brucella melitensis* (goats), and *Brucella canis* (dogs). *Brucella* enters the body by way of the skin, digestive tract, or respiratory tract, following which it may enter the blood and lymphatics. It is an intracellular pathogen that multiplies inside phagocytes to eventually cause bacteremia (bacterial blood infiltration). Symptoms include fever, sweats, malaise, anorexia, headache, myalgia, and back pain. In the undulant form (<1 year from illness onset), symptoms include undulant fevers, arthritis, with a possible neurologic manifestation in a small number of cases. In the chronic form, symptoms can include chronic fatigue syndrome with accompanying depression and eventual arthritis. Afflicted individuals are successfully treated with streptomycin or erythromycin.

Francisella

Francisella tularensis is a small, gram-negative, aerobic bacillus. The two main serotypes are Jellison types A and B. Type A is the more virulent form; infection through tick bite or direct contact will lead to tularemia. *F. tularensis*, also referred to as *Pasteurella tularensis*, causes sudden fever, chills, headaches, diarrhea, muscle aches, joint pain, dry cough, and progressive weakness. The disease also can be contracted by ingestion or inhalation. Tularemia occurs in six different forms including typhoidal, pneumonic, oculoglandular, oropharyngeal, ulceroglandular, and glandular. Treatment includes a regimen of streptomycin or gentamycin.

Bartonella

Bartonella henselae is a fastidious, gram-negative bacterium that is the cause of many diseases such as bacillary angiomatosis, visceral peliosis, septicemia, endocarditis, and cat-scratch disease. The most common symptoms are persisting fever lasting up to 8 weeks, abdominal pain, and lesions around sites of infection. Aminoglycosides and rifampin are effective and bactericidal, whereas β-lactams are ineffective in treatment.

Vibrio

The *Vibrio* genus contains motile, gram-negative bacteria that are obligate aerobes. They are comma-shaped rods with a single polar flagellum, facultative anaerobes that are oxidase-positive. Although *Vibrio* spp are noninvasive pathogens, they cause severe diarrheal illness and thousands of deaths annually. The organisms are waterborne and are transmitted to humans through ingestion of infected water or through fecal transmission.

Vibrio cholerae is the causative agent of cholera, characterized by severe diarrhea with a rice-water color and consistency. Sixty percent of cholera deaths are due to dehydration. Ingested organisms descend to the intestinal tract, bind to epithelium, and subsequently release an exotoxin (choleragen) (Fig. 12-5), causing water to passively flow out of cells. It is critical to replace fluids and electrolytes when treating cholera patients. *V. cholerae* is susceptible to administration of doxycycline or tetracycline, as are other members of this species. *Vibrio parahaemolyticus* is another species that causes diarrhea as well as cramps, nausea, and fever. The disease is transmitted by eating infected seafood and is self-limiting to about 3 days. *Vibrio vulnificus* and *Vibrio parahaemolyticus* may also be contracted from contaminated seafood. Unlike other *Vibrio* spp, *V. vulnificus* is invasive and able to enter the bloodstream through the epithelium of the gut. Fever, vomiting, and chills are the symptoms; wound infections can occur with resulting cellulitis or ulcer formations.

●●● CAMPYLOBACTER AND HELICOBACTER

Two groups of gram-negative organisms, *Campylobacter* and *Helicobacter*, may be found residing in gut tissue. Both are curved or spiral-shaped and are genetically related. Both are motile and catalase-positive. Organisms of the genus *Campylobacter* are gram-negative microaerophiles that cause diarrhea. They achieve cell motility by way of polar flagella. *Campylobacter jejuni* causes gastroenteritis and is usually acquired by eating undercooked food or drinking contaminated milk or water. Symptoms of infection are fever, cramps, and bloody diarrhea, which is caused by penetration of the lining of the small intestine. It can be treated with antibiotics (erythromycin) but is usually self-limited.

Helicobacter spp also are gram-negative, microaerophilic organisms. *Helicobacter pylori* is a spiral-shaped bacterium that is found in the gastric mucus layer or adherent to the epithelial lining of the stomach. *H. pylori* causes more than 90% of duodenal ulcers and up to 80% of gastric ulcers. The mechanisms of pathogenesis for ulceration remain incompletely defined. The organism characteristically produces a urease that generates ammonia and CO_2. Infected patients can be treated with an antacid as well as tetracycline to treat the ulcers and inhibit the growth of the organism.

●●● NONFERMENTERS

The nonfermenters are gram-negative rods that either do not ferment glucose for energy or do not use glucose at all. *Pseudomonas* and *Acinetobacter* spp fall into this category. Pseudomonads are motile organisms that utilize glucose oxidatively. *Pseudomonas* comprises five groups based on ribosomal RNA (rRNA)/DNA homology. These bacteria are often encountered in hospital settings and are a major source of nosocomial infections. Clinically, they are resistant to most antibiotics and capable of surviving in harsh conditions. Both organisms target immunocompromised individuals, burn victims, and individuals on respirators or with indwelling catheters. Pseudomonads produce an alginate slime layer that is resistant to phagocytosis. They readily colonize the lungs of cystic fibrosis patients, increasing the mortality rate of these individuals. Infection may occur in multiple tissues, leading to urinary tract infections, sepsis, pneumonia, and pharyngitis.

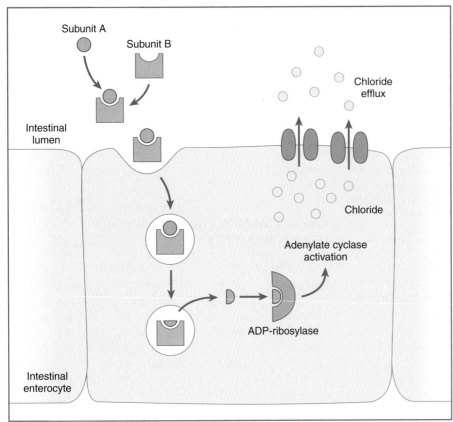

Subunit A

Subunit B

Intestinal
lumen

Chloride
efflux

Chloride

Adenylate cyclase
activation

ADP-ribosylase

Intestinal
enterocyte

Figure 12-5. Pathogenesis of *Vibrio cholerae*. *V. cholerae* organisms adhere to the intestinal microvilli upon which cholera toxin is secreted. The toxin contains two subunits (A and B); the B subunit binds to gangliosides on epithelial cell surfaces allowing internalization of the A subunit. B subunits provide a hydrophobic channel through which A penetrates, following which the A subunit catalyses ADP-ribosylation to activate adenylate cyclase in cell membranes of gut epithelium. The end result is massive secretion of ions and water into the gut lumen with resultant dehydration.

Pseudomonas

Pseudomonas aeruginosa is commonly isolated from clinical specimens (wound, burn, and urinary tract infections). It may be found widely distributed in soil and water. Its pathogenicity involves bacterial attachment and colonization, followed by local invasion, and dissemination with systemic disease. A surface lipopolysaccharide layer assists in adherence to host tissues and prevents leukocytes from ingesting and lysing the organism. Lipases and exotoxins then proceed to destroy host cell tissue. In healthy children, diseases are limited primarily to those associated with attachment and local infection, e.g., otitis externa, UTIs, dermatitis, and cellulitis. In immunocompromised hosts and neonates who do not have a fully competent immune response, infection may appear as a disseminated infection, e.g., pneumonia, endocarditis, peritonitis, meningitis, and overwhelming septicemia.

P. aeruginosa and *Pseudomonas maltophilia* account for 80% of opportunistic infections by pseudomonads. *Burkholderia (Pseudomonas) cepacia* is a related opportunistic pathogen of cystic fibrosis patients that can be distinguished from *Pseudomonas* spp because it is lysine-positive. The spread of pseudomonas is best controlled by cleaning and disinfecting medical equipment. Pseudomonads typically are resistant to multiple therapeutic and antimicrobial agents; therefore, antibiotic susceptibility testing of clinical isolates is mandatory. In general, the combination of gentamicin and carbenicillin can be effective in treatment of acute infections.

Acinetobacter

Acinetobacter spp are oxidase-negative, nonmotile bacteria. They appear as gram-negative coccobacilli when viewed microscopically. *Acinetobacter* poses little risk to healthy people; individuals with weakened immune systems, chronic lung disease, or diabetes may be more susceptible to infection. *Acinetobacter baumannii* accounts for about 80% of reported infections and is linked to hospital-acquired infections of the skin and open wounds. In addition, *A. baumannii* is a major agent leading to pneumonia and meningitis. *Acinetobacter lwoffi* is the causative agent for the majority of reported meningitis caused by *Acinetobacter*. Owing to high resistance to multiple antibiotics, a combination of aminoglycoside and a second agent is usually recommended for treatment.

Although not of the same genus, *Stenotrophomonas maltophilia* (formerly known as *Xanthomonas maltophilia*) is similar to the pseudomonads. This motile bacterium is a cause of nosocomial infections in immunocompromised patients. *Flavobacterium* spp are ubiquitous organisms that can cause infection in premature infants and immunocompromised individuals. Most species metabolize glucose oxidatively; all species are motile and oxidase-positive. Of clinical importance, *Flavobacterium meningosepticum* causes neonatal meningitis and is typically penicillin resistant.

●●● ANAEROBIC GRAM-NEGATIVE BACILLI

Bacteroides

Bacteroides spp are anaerobic bacteria that inhabit the digestive tract; interestingly, 50% of fecal matter is composed of *Bacteroides fragilis* cells! *Bacteroides* organisms are the anaerobic counterpart of *E. coli*. They grow well on blood agar. Microscopically, they appear to contain large vacuoles similar in appearance to spores. *Bacteroides* spp produce a very large capsule but are not spore-forming. They do not possess an endotoxin in their cell membrane, which limits their pathogenicity. Infection occurs after severe trauma to the gut and abdominal region, resulting in abscess formation with accompanying fever. Antibiotic treatment consists of metronidazole or clindamycin.

Fusobacterium

Fusobacterium organisms are anaerobic, gram-negative bacilli that are similar to certain *Bacteroides* spp. They appear as spindle-shaped cells with sharp ends. Both reside in the gut but are capable of causing serious infection. *Fusobacterium* spp, the most common of which is *Fusobacterium nucleatum*, are associated with pleuropulmonary infections and congestion exhibited as sinusitis. They are also capable of causing infection in the oral cavity (the mouth) and may be a major cause of gingivitis.

●●● SPIROCHETES

Spirochetes are long, slender bacteria, usually only a fraction of a micron in diameter but anywhere from 5 to 250 microns long. The best known spirochetes of clinical importance are those which cause disease, including syphilis and Lyme disease.

Treponema

Treponema pallidum is the causative organism of syphilis. It is a motile spirochete that is generally acquired by close sexual contact, entering host tissue by breaches in squamous or columnar epithelium. Disease is marked by a primary chancre (an area of ulceration and inflammation) seen in genital areas, which manifests soon after the primary infection. Progression to secondary and tertiary syphilis is marked by maculopapular rashes and eventual granulomatous response with CNS involvement. Nonvenereal treponemal diseases include pinta, caused by *Treponema carateum*, and disfiguring yaws, caused by *Treponema pallidum* subsp *pertenue*.

Borrelia

Borrelia burgdorferi is the spirochete that causes Lyme disease. In contrast to *T. pallidum*, *Borrelia* has a unique nucleus

PATHOLOGY

Erythema Migrans

Erythema migrans (also called erythema chronicum migrans) is the skin lesion that develops at the site of a bite from a deer tick infected with borreliosis. The early lesion is characterized by an expanding area of red rash, often with a pale center ("bulls-eye") at the site of the tick bite, indicative of early signs of Lyme disease.

containing a linear chromosome and linear plasmids. *Borrelia* is transmitted by tick bites (*Ixodes*) during blood feeding. Early indications of Lyme disease are a distinctive skin lesion, called erythema migrans. If it is left untreated, an erosive arthritis can occur similar to rheumatoid arthritis, and eventual chronic progressive encephalitis and encephalomyelitis. A number of other *Borrelia* spp can cause endemic relapsing fever, with causative agents including *Borrelia duttonii*, *Borrelia hermsii*, and *Borrelia dugesi*.

●●● OBLIGATE INTRACELLULAR PATHOGENS

Chlamydia

Obligate intracellular pathogens of clinical importance include the *Chlamydia* and *Rickettsia* spp. *Chlamydia* are small, obligate, intracellular parasites that were once considered to be viruses. The family Chlamydiaceae consists of one genus *Chlamydia* with three species that cause human disease. *Chlamydia trachomatis* can cause urogenital infections, trachoma, conjunctivitis, pneumonia, and lymphogranuloma venereum (LGV). *Chlamydia pneumoniae* can cause bronchitis, sinusitis and pneumonia. *Chlamydia psittaci* can cause pneumonia (psittacosis). *Chlamydia* spp have an inner and outer membrane and a glycolipid but not a peptidoglycan layer. They are unable to make their own ATP and thus are energy parasites. The structure of all three species is similar. The infectious agent is the elementary body form (EB), which is characterized by a rigid outer membrane that is extensively cross-linked by disulfide bonds. The elementary bodies bind to receptors on host epithelial cells to initiate infection (Fig. 12-6). Metabolically active, replicating intracellular forms are referred to as reticulate bodies (RBs). RBs possess a fragile membrane lacking the extensive disulfide bonds characteristic of the EB. Human infectious biovars have been subdivided into serovars (serologic variants) that differ in major outer membrane proteins. The *C. trachomatis* serovars A, B, and C are associated with ocular disease; serovars D through K are associated with conjunctivitis, urethritis, cervicitis, and pneumonia; and serovars L1, L2, and L3 are associated with lymphogranuloma venereum. *C. pneumoniae* is the causative agent of an atypical pneumonia similar to that caused by *Mycoplasma pneumoniae*. The organism is transmitted person-to-person

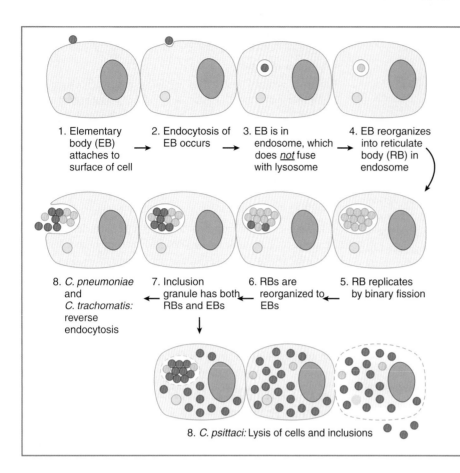

Figure 12-6. Chlamydial developmental cycle. Infectious elementary bodies (EB) bind to receptors on susceptible epithelial cells and are internalized. Inside the host cell endosomes, reorganization into the reticulate body (RB) form occurs. This is accompanied by inhibition of the fusion of endosomes with lysosomes to limit intracellular killing. RBs replicate by binary fission and finally reorganize into rigid EBs; inclusions containing up to 500 progeny are extruded by reverse endocytosis or by cell death and subsequent cell lysis.

by respiratory droplets. For all the *Chlamydia*, effective treatment includes tetracyclines, erythromycin, or sulfonamides.

Rickettsia, Ehrlichia, and Coxiella

The genera *Rickettsia*, *Ehrlichia*, and *Coxiella* are a diverse collection of gram-negative, obligate, intracellular bacteria found in arthropod vectors (ixodid ticks, lice, and fleas). They are considered zoonotic pathogens. They infect white blood cells, causing blood-borne, disseminated infections of endothelium and vascular smooth muscle. *Rickettsia rickettsii* causes Rocky Mountain spotted fever and a form of rickettsialpox. *Ehrlichia* spp cause ehrlichioses. *Coxiella* spp (*Coxiella burnetii*) cause Q fever that manifests as an acute febrile illness with pneumonia or as a chronic infection with accompanying endocarditis. All of these species are sensitive to doxycycline and tetracycline.

●●● ACID-FAST ORGANISMS

A number of clinically relevant organisms are described as "acid-fast" owing to their staining properties with carbolfuchsin stain (Ziehl-Neelsen stain); only acid-fast organisms retain the stain following treatment with an acid alcohol. A brilliant red coloration results owing to retention of carbolfuchsin within the cell membrane. Although the exact molecular mechanism for dye retention is unknown, this group of organisms is characterized by a high content of

mycolic acids within cellular membranes. Of these organisms, the mycobacteria are of major clinical relevance with nearly one-third of the world's population infected. *Nocardia* spp and intestinal Coccidia also belong to this group; pathologic manifestations of infection caused by these organisms are discussed.

Mycobacterium

As discussed in Chapter 10, organisms that are the causative agents of tuberculosis and leprosy have evolved to inhibit normal macrophage killing mechanisms (e.g., phagosome-lysosome fusion) and survive within the "disarmed" professional phagocyte. This leads to development of hypersensitive pathologies, established to contain a central nidus of infection. Mycobacteria are nonmotile, slow-growing, rod-shaped organisms that are obligate aerobes. They have a cell envelope with a high lipid content and contain complex, long-chain fatty acids (mycolic acids) that are found otherwise only in *Nocardia* and *Corynebacterium*. Mycobacteria are catalase-positive, with the exception of nonpathogenic *Mycobacterium kansasii* and isoniazid (INH)–resistant *Mycobacterium tuberculosis*.

Mycobacterium tuberculosis

M. tuberculosis (MTB) is a major health concern, with an estimated 8.4 million new cases a year and 2 to 3 million deaths worldwide. The organism is acquired through inhalation of aerosolized infected droplets. It has an extremely slow growth rate (doubling time of 18 hours), and a cell envelope that is rich in waxes and lipids, especially mycolic acids that are covalently linked to arabinogalactans (Fig. 12-7). Once inside the host, the organism is engulfed by macrophages, stimulating responses leading to exudative (pneumonia-like) or granulomatous lesions. The granulomatous lesions are characterized by giant multinucleated cells, surrounded by lymphocytes, forming the basis of a tubercle. Necrotic events occur as the organisms persist, leaving a caseous center to the granulomatous response. Eventual erosion of lesions into bronchial airways leads to spread of disease. Resolution may occur, leaving remnant fibrotic and calcified lesions, which are referred to as Ghon complexes. Most individuals will successfully contain organisms. However, immunocompromised individuals (due to HIV infection, malnutrition, old age, or immunosuppression) can undergo reactivation events, typically with evidence of disseminated infection and reseeding of organisms to apical lung tissue.

Exposure to mycobacterial surface antigens leads to responses that can easily be detected using the tuberculin skin test, functionally detecting an inducible delayed-type hypersensitive response. Small amounts of purified protein derivative (PPD; Mantoux test) are injected intradermally; induration occurring within 24 hours signifies positive exposure to organisms. Because of the slow growth of the

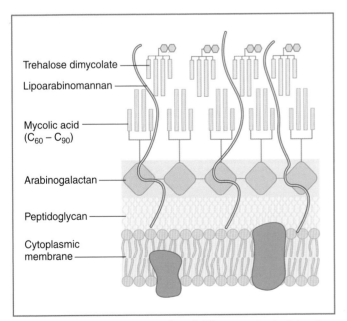

Figure 12-7. Mycobacterial cell wall. The mycobacterial cell envelope is rich in waxes and lipids, especially mycolic acids, which are covalently linked to arabinogalactans. The unique long-chain mycolic acid trehalose 6,6′-dimycolate (C_{60}–C_{90}) is responsible for "cording" seen with virulent strains, giving colonies a serpentine morphology. Mycolic acids form an asymmetric lipid bilayer with shorter chain glycerophospholipids. The cell envelope also contains peptidoglycan and has a complex glycolipid structure forming the outermost layer, which sits atop the peptidoglycan and lipid bilayer of the cytoplasmic membrane. Other important components include lipoarabinomannan and arabinogalactan.

Labels in figure:
Trehalose dimycolate
Lipoarabinomannan
Mycolic acid (C_{60} – C_{90})
Arabinogalactan
Peptidoglycan
Cytoplasmic membrane

organisms and the presence of the waxy cell envelope, therapeutics to combat infection must be given for long periods. It is typical to administer 6 months of therapy with a first-line antituberculosis agent, such as INH, rifampin, pyrazinamide, streptomycin, or ethambutol. In cases of drug resistance, a second-line antituberculosis drug may also be prescribed, such as para-aminosalicylic acid (PAS), rifabutin, ethionamide, kanamycin, or a fluoroquinolone.

Atypical Mycobacteria

The atypical mycobacteria include *M. kansasii*, which causes a lung disease clinically resembling MTB, especially in individuals with preexisting lung conditions. *Mycobacterium marinum* causes "swimming pool granulomas" and abscesses. *Mycobacterium avium-intracellulare* complex (MAC) is pleomorphic, with multiple disease-causing serovars included in this group. MAC infections typically cause pulmonary disease similar to MTB in the immunocompromised host; disseminated infection is typical in individuals with complicating HIV infections. *Mycobacterium fortuitum* and *Mycobacterium chelonei* are saprophytes that rarely cause disease; however, infections have been reported in individuals with joint replacements.

Mycobacterium leprae

M. leprae causes leprosy, which is also known as Hansen's disease. The optimal temperature for growth is lower than core body temperature, so it grows on skin and superficial nerves, infecting macrophages and Schwann cells. *M. leprae* has resisted efforts for growth in culture and thus is difficult to study. There are two clinical spectra of disease—tuberculoid and lepromatous leprosy—based on immune function and host response. The high resistance of tuberculoid leprosy is associated with cellular response and formation of prominent granulomatous lesions. Delayed hypersensitivity skin tests are intact, and there is predominant hyperplasia of the lymph nodes. Lepromatous leprosy is associated with the accumulation of highly activated, "foamy" macrophages filled with viable organisms. Delayed hypersensitivity skin tests are depressed; the levels of antibodies are high and vascular lesions occur (erythema nodosum leprosum). Borderline leprosy has intermediate findings. Clinically, lepromatous leprosy is characterized by symmetric skin nodules, plaques, and loss of eyelashes and body hair. Loss of digits in leprosy is due to trauma and secondary infection. Treatment for leprosy consists of dapsone and clofazimine.

Nocardia

Respiratory infection due to *Nocardia* may occur through inhalation, whereas primary cutaneous disease results from soil contamination of wounds. Most cases present as an invasive pulmonary disorder with potential for disseminated disease that may lead to brain abscess; however, 20% of cases present as cellulitis. *Nocardia asteroides* is the major organism accounting for infections, although other pathogenic species have been identified, including *Nocardia farcinica*, *Nocardia nova*, *Nocardia transvalensis*, *Nocardia brasiliensis*, and *Nocardia pseudobrasiliensis*.

Acid-Fast Intestinal Coccidia

Three intestinal coccidia infecting humans stain acid-fast and should be considered unicellular protozoa. They are *Cryptosporidium parvum*, *Cyclospora cayetanensis*, and *Isospora belli*. *C. parvum* is the etiologic agent of diarrheal disease (cryptosporidiosis) caused by members of the genus *Cryptosporidium*. The most common symptom of cryptosporidiosis is watery diarrhea, with accompanying dehydration, weight loss, stomach cramps or pain, fever, nausea, and vomiting. *Cryptosporidium* is resistant to chlorine and can be spread in pool water. *Cryptosporidium cayetanensis* is the agent causing cyclosporiasis. *Cyclospora* infects the small intestine (bowel), resulting in watery diarrhea with frequent, sometimes explosive, bowel movements. The agent for isosporiasis, *Isospora belli*, infects epithelial cells of the small intestine and is the least common of the three intestinal coccidia.

●●● MYCOPLASMA

Mycoplasma pneumoniae is a small (0.3 μm diameter), wall-less organism that is transmitted through aerosolized droplets. *Mycoplasma* binds firmly to respiratory epithelium; it is the causative agent of nonviral atypical pneumonia symptomatically characterized by sore throat, headache, myalgia, and whitish, nonbloody sputum. Infection with *M. pneumoniae* can lead to autoantibody production (usually IgM isotypes), producing cross-reactive antibodies directed against red cell antigens. The autoantibodies are referred to as cold agglutinins and cause a reactive, autoimmune, hemolytic disease. Because *Mycoplasma* has no cell wall, agents such as penicillin and cephalosporins are not effective.

Basic Virology

13

CONTENTS

Viruses are small entities (20–300 nm) whose genomes replicate inside cells using host cellular machinery to create progeny virions (virus particles). On its own, a virus may be considered an inert biochemical complex of macromolecules, since it cannot replicate outside a living cell. However, viruses are known to infect all living organisms, and a broad variety of viruses contribute to human disease.

KEY POINTS ABOUT VIRUSES

- Viruses are entities whose genomes replicate inside cells using host cellular machinery to create progeny virions (virus particles) that can transfer the genome to other cells.

- A broad variety of viruses are of high medical significance and contribute to manifestations of human disease.

●●● VIRAL CLASSIFICATION AND STRUCTURE

Historically, viruses were named according to common pathogenic properties, organ tropism, and modes of transmission. Viral groups are classified based upon viral host range, particle morphology, and genome type. Viral hosts represent species from all classes of cellular organisms; prokaryotes (including the Archaea and Bacteria), eukaryotes (including algae, plants, protozoa, and fungi), and complex invertebrates and vertebrates. Indeed, viruses can cross phyla; e.g., different members of Poxviridae can infect vertebrates and insects.

Virion structure varies among different viral groups, yet all virus particles are enclosed by a capsid structure that surrounds the viral genome. Icosahedral symmetry is the preferred capsid morphology (Fig. 13-1). The capsid is a protein shell composed of repeating subunits, or protomers (also referred to as capsomeres). The capsid together with the enclosed nucleic acid is called the nucleocapsid. The term *virion* denotes the complete infective virus particle. Many viruses demonstrate the classic capsid polyhedron structure of 20 equilateral triangular faces and 12 vertices, which define axes of fivefold rotational symmetry. However, alternative virion morphologies exist. Some viruses have a helical nucleocapsid, consisting of a helical array of capsid proteins composed of identical protomers wrapped around a filament of nucleic acid. Thus, for these viruses, such as myxoviruses (e.g., tobacco mosaic virus), the length of the helical nucleocapsid is determined by the length of the nucleic acid.

Other virus families have an outer envelope consisting of a lipid bilayer surrounding the viral capsid. Such viral envelopes are derived in part from modified host cell membranes during particle formation and release (budding) from the infected cell. The exterior of the bilayer is studded with glycosylated (*trans*) membrane proteins, revealed as glycoprotein spikes or knobs. Both the outer capsid and envelope proteins of viruses are glycosylated and are important in determining the host range and antigenic composition of the virion.

KEY POINTS ABOUT VIRAL CLASSIFICATION AND STRUCTURE

- Icosahedral symmetry is the preferred status for organization of virus structure subunits (protomers) making up the capsid protein shell.

- Other structural forms exist, yet they all share commonality in packaging of genetic material (DNA or RNA) for delivery to host cells upon infection.

●●● VIRAL GENETIC MATERIAL: RNA OR DNA

Each virus carries within the protective capsid a nucleic acid–based blueprint for replication of infectious virus particles (virions). Once a virus has invaded a cell, it is able to direct the host cell machinery to synthesize new progeny.

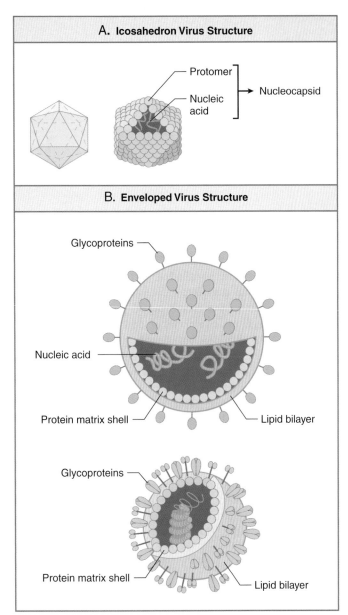

A. Icosahedron Virus Structure

Protomer
Nucleic acid
Nucleocapsid

B. Enveloped Virus Structure

Glycoproteins
Nucleic acid
Protein matrix shell
Lipid bilayer

Glycoproteins
Protein matrix shell
Lipid bilayer

Figure 13-1. Basic virus structure. The basic virus structure is an icosahedron having 20 equilateral triangular faces and 12 vertices. Lines through opposite vertices define axes of fivefold rotational symmetry with structural features repeating five times within each complete rotation about any axis (**A**). A nucleocapsid contains DNA or RNA encapsulated within a capsid composed of protomer subunits. Enveloped virions (**B**) support an outer lipid bilayer studded with transmembrane glycoprotein spikes. Other forms of viral structure exist, such as those with helical nucleocapsid symmetry in which size of the virus is dictated by the length of nucleic acid core (not shown).

The viral genome may be composed of RNA or DNA, single- or double-stranded. Encoded proteins may be nonstructural, such as nucleic acid polymerases required for replication of genetic material, or structural (those proteins necessary for assembly of new infectious virions). However, all viruses lack the genetic information encoding proteins necessary to generate metabolic energy or protein synthesis. The viral genome (DNA or RNA) rarely codes for more than the few proteins necessary for replication or physical structure.

Viruses as a group are the only class of organisms with subspecies that keep RNA as their sole genetic material. Likewise, they are the only group of self-replicating organisms with subspecies that utilize single-stranded DNA as genomic content. Multiple forms of virus genomes are found in virions infecting human cells (Fig. 13-2).

●●● STRATEGIES FOR INFECTIVITY AND REPLICATION

The first stage of viral infection and subsequent replication involves entry into the host cell (Fig. 13-3). The host cell phenotype has a great deal of influence on the strategy the virus uses to gain access; in turn, specific virus types may employ different strategies to gain access to the same cell type. In general, the steps involve attachment and penetration, uncoating of the virus genome, and synthesis of early proteins (enzymes involved in viral replication) followed by synthesis of late proteins or structural components required for assembly and release of the infectious virion.

Viral entry into the cell is usually a passive reaction that does not require energy on the part of the virus. Naked viral particles may enter by membrane translocation, in which the entire virus crosses the cell border intact (pinocytosis). Alternatively, the naked particle binds to cell surface receptors and subsequent invagination occurs by either clathrin-mediated endocytosis (e.g., Adenoviridae) or other endocytic mechanisms such as interaction with caveolae or lipid rafts. A naked viral particle may also bind to the cell surface and inject genomic material into the host cell, without complete cellular penetration of the invading virion. Enveloped viruses must enter host cells using mechanisms of membrane fusion, either via receptor-mediated endocytosis or through fusion of viral and host membranes, followed by injection of genomic material into the host cell cytoplasm (e.g., HIV-1 and HIV-2). In all cases, the critical component is the release of the viral genome from its protective capsid so that it can be transcribed to form new progeny virions.

In many cases, viral genetic material undergoes translation using host cellular machinery prior to viral genome replication (the exception being retroviruses and negative-sense

BIOCHEMISTRY

Clathrin-Mediated Endocytosis

Receptor-mediated endocytosis is a complex phenomenon in which binding of large extracellular molecules, such as viruses, to receptors on the cell membrane triggers assembly of clathrin triskelions. Specific clathrin adapter complexes are involved in transport across the membrane, resulting in endosomal compartment formation.

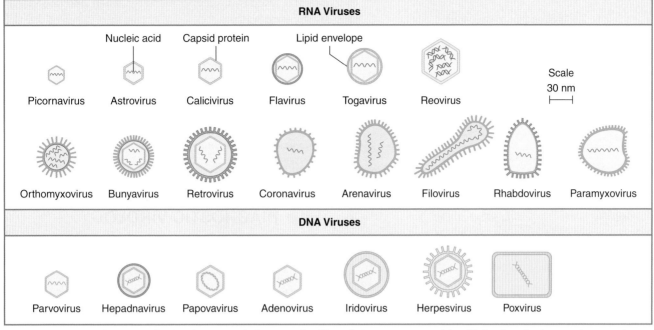

Figure 13-2. Virus families infecting humans. At least 21 families of viruses are capable of infecting the human host and are distinguished by the presence of an envelope or characteristic capsid and internal nucleic acid genomic content.

RNA viruses). The first proteins generated are usually non-structural DNA or RNA polymerases. Nucleic acid replication produces new viral genomes for incorporation into progeny virions. In general, DNA viruses replicate mainly in the nucleus and RNA viruses mainly in the cytoplasm, but there are exceptions (e.g., poxviruses contain DNA but replicate in the cytoplasm). Retroviruses are a special category of RNA viruses that require reverse transcription of their single-stranded RNA genome to a double-stranded DNA inter-mediate, which is then integrated into the host cell genome before viral replication can take place. Retroviruses not only encode a reverse transcriptase enzyme as part of the virion but also package it into newly formed virions.

The next set of proteins to be transcribed are structural in nature, including capsid protomers and scaffolding proteins that are required for assembly of the virion together with the newly replicated viral nucleic acid. Assembly of viral nucleo-capsids can take place in either the nucleus (herpesvirus, adenovirus), cytoplasm (poliovirus), or cell surface (influenza). Diagnostic inclusions, sometimes visible by light microscopy, are the result of virions accumulating at the sites of assembly. The final stage of replication results in the release of newly formed virions from the host cell. This may occur by budding from the cell surface (enveloped viruses) or via host cellular secretory pathways in which Golgi-derived vesicles are transported to the cell surface. In nonenveloped viruses, host cells are destroyed, with consequent release of infectious virions upon cell lysis.

The Baltimore classification of viruses establishes seven groupings according to genome types and replication strategies (Table 13-1).

KEY POINTS ABOUT STRATEGIES FOR INFECTIVITY AND REPLICATION

- Initiation of viral replication begins with attachment and entry of viral particles into host cells, followed by replication of genetic material and production of assisting proteins (polymerases and structural proteins) required for assembly of virions with mature nucleocapsids.

- Newly formed virions are released from the host cells by assembly at the cell surface, via budding, or by lysis of the host cell.

- Multiple and diverse replication strategies are used, depending upon the type and class of genetic material contained within the virus entity.

●●● VIRAL DISEASE PATTERNS AND PATHOGENESIS

Virus-induced pathology is the result of direct viral action leading to host cell death and tissue damage with subsequent sequelae. Almost all naked (nonenveloped) viruses produce acute infections in this manner, owing to cell lysis during replication and spread of infection to surrounding host cells. However, pathologic damage is often a result of an active immune response to viral antigens and epitopes presented on the surface of infected cells (Fig. 13-4). This becomes especially apparent in chronic infections when persistent virus production allows vigorous development of cellular (T_H and CTL generation) and humoral (B cells with specific antiviral antibodies) responses. In the case of latent infections, short periods of active viral replication are kept in check by active

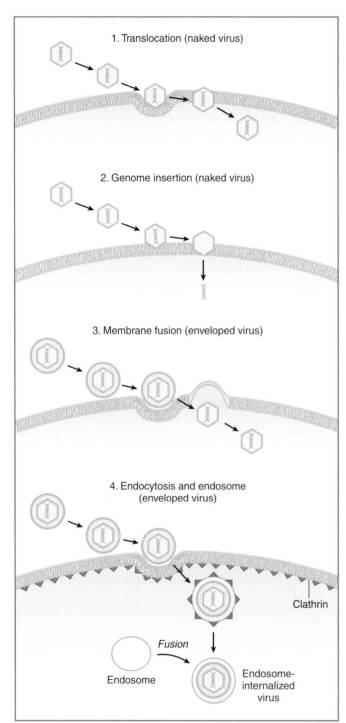

1. Translocation (naked virus)

2. Genome insertion (naked virus)

3. Membrane fusion (enveloped virus)

4. Endocytosis and endosome
(enveloped virus)

Clathrin

Fusion

Endosome

Endosome-internalized virus

Figure 13-3. Mechanisms of viral infection of host cells. Viruses enter host cells following attachment by multiple means including (1) translocation, in which virus crosses membranes intact; (2) genome insertion, in which attached viruses inject genetic material directly into cytoplasm; (3) membrane fusion, in which genomic contents of virus are dumped into the host cell cytoplasm; and (4) endocytosis dictated by surface receptor binding and clathrin-mediated transport, sometimes leading to fusion into intracellular endosomes.

immune responses, only to reemerge when immune system surveillance wanes.

KEY POINTS ABOUT VIRAL DISEASE PATTERNS AND PATHOGENESIS

- Pathology associated with viral infections is directly linked to viral cell tropism and mechanism of associated replication.

- Damage to surrounding tissue may be a direct result of the immune response and attempts to limit viral replication and spread.

●●● DIAGNOSTIC VIROLOGY

The large number of possible viral agents that produce a given disease or pathology precludes the use of one simple test as diagnostic for identification. Rather, laboratory diagnosis is usually performed under the assumption of clinical disease spectrum, relying on symptoms and epidemiologic data (Fig. 13-5). Clinical observations alone are at times sufficient for diagnosis, allowing for clear therapeutic intervention prior to verification of virus identity. The identification of a virus from a clinical specimen relies on general characteristics such as the ability to replicate or produce certain phenotypes in cell culture. In vitro propagation in tissue culture can determine level of infection. Typically, viral growth in tissue culture produces a cytopathogenic effect (CPE), which may be visualized as a plaque or vacancy within a monolayer of cells. Infected cells may be further fixed and stained; immunohistochemical methods can be used to determine the presence of characteristic and diagnostic inclusions (or inclusion bodies) in cytoplasm or in the nucleus. Along with these diagnostic tools, specificity may be obtained by using antibodies to neutralize the viral agent and confirm its identification. Incubation of infected cells with neutralizing antibodies will result in reduction of growth of the virus and subsequent reduction in the number of plaques formed.

Serologic tests are useful to confirm induced responses to viral antigens. Serum collected from infected individuals may be assessed for antibody response using the enzyme-linked immunosorbent assay (ELISA). Enzyme immunoassays, also known as solid-phase immunoassays, are designed to detect antibodies through secondary production of an enzyme-triggered color change. ELISAs are useful in detecting and quantifying the presence of viral agents in clinical specimens (blood, vaginal swabs, and feces). Use of specific antibodies immobilized to a solid-phase also allows capture of pathogens for diagnostic quantitation to known standards.

Identification of viral agents in clinical specimens also may be performed using highly sensitive genetic tools. RNA or DNA can be extracted and sequences probed by hybridization techniques. If the agent is already identified, analysis can also be accomplished by use of polymerase chain reaction (PCR) or reverse-transcriptase PCR (RT-PCR) to specifically amplify sequences unique to the viral agent under consid-

TABLE 13-1. Different Classes of Viruses Grouped According to Replication Strategy (Baltimore Classification)

Class	Genome Type	Replication Strategy	Examples of Genus Infecting Human Cells
I	dsDNA	Semiconservative method using bidirectional replication forks from a single origin	Poxvirus Herpesvirus Adenovirus Papovavirus
II	ssDNA	Formation of a replicative from double-stranded DNA intermediate	Parvovirus
III	dsRNA replicating via (+) RNA	Conservative mechanism in which input RNA is transcribed to mRNA	Reovirus
IV	ssRNA (+) sense genomes	Synthesis of (−) sense RNA on a (+) sense template	Coronavirus Flavivirus Astrovirus Picornavirus
V	ssRNA (−) sense genomes	Begins with transcription by virion-associated RNA-dependent RNA polymerase	Arenavirus Orthomyxovirus Paramyxovirus Rhabdovirus
VI	Diploid ssRNA	Via a dsDNA, longer-than-genome-length intermediate (provirus), which is integrated covalently into host cell chromosomal DNA	Retrovirus
VII	dsDNA	Via gapped or nicked circular dsDNA genomes that replicate via longer-than-genome-length messenger-sense ssRNA intermediates	Hepadnavirus

(+), Sense strand; (−), antisense strand.

eration. However, in some instances, this task is difficult or impossible because of atypical clinical presentation or histopathologic features. Molecular diagnostics using DNA microarrays, or gene chip arrays, offer the promise of precise, objective, and systematic virus classification from clinically obtained specimens. In addition, diagnostic gene chip arrays that carry sequences of major clinically relevant viral pathogens will allow for extremely rapid screening of small diagnostic samples.

●●● THERAPY AND PROPHYLAXIS FOR VIRAL INFECTIONS

Therapy against viral infection makes use of chemotherapeutic agents that are effective to control infection and disease. Virucides, such as detergents, chloroform, and UV light, utilize general mechanisms to limit environmental spread of viruses. This is especially effective at reducing levels of enveloped organisms that are sensitive because of their bilipid envelope. Antiviral agents are more specific and include molecules that target receptors for cell attachment or that inhibit viral penetration, uncoating of the viral genome, or viral replication. Inhibition of replication may occur at multiple stages; agents may be directed against macromolecular synthesis and inhibit transcription, translation, or posttranslational modification (e.g., protease inhibitors). The majority of clinically available antiviral agents target nucleic

acid synthesis and limit viral replication rather than completely eliminating organisms (virustatic vs. virucidal). Problems associated with host toxicity limit the use of virucidal agents in many instances. An additional concern is the selective pressure associated with prolonged use of antiviral agents that allows mutants to arise which are no longer susceptible to drug action.

Another class of antiviral agents includes those that function as immunomodulators to improve host response to combat infection. These antivirals do not directly attack the specific pathogen, but rather they globally stimulate host immune responses. Interferons (IFNs) were first defined as glycoproteins that interfere with viral replication through degradation of viral mRNA. Most nucleated cells make

---

PHARMACOLOGY

Antiviral Agents: HAART (Highly Active Antiretroviral Therapy)

HAART holds great promise to limit HIV infection by means of agents that are terminal nucleoside analogs, non-nucleoside reverse transcriptase inhibitors, and viral protease inhibitors. Zidovudine was the first FDA-approved antiretroviral and is an analog of thymidine that works as a nucleoside analog reverse transcriptase inhibitor (NARTI).

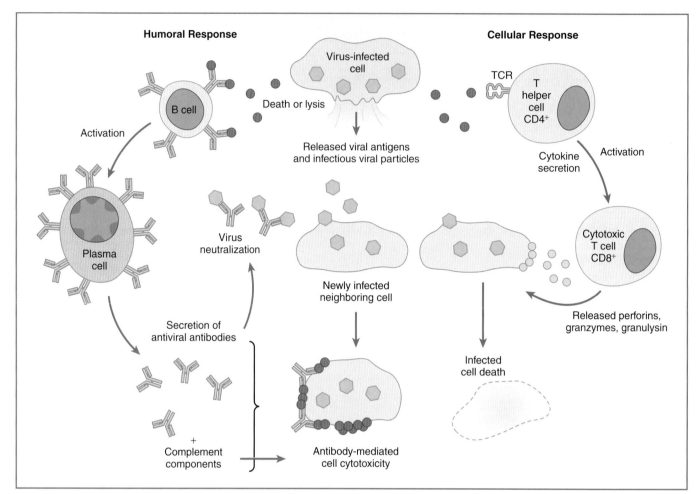

Humoral Response

Cellular Response

Virus-infected cell

B cell

Death or lysis

TCR

T helper cell CD4+

Activation

Released viral antigens and infectious viral particles

Cytokine secretion

Activation

Virus neutralization

Plasma cell

Secretion of antiviral antibodies

Newly infected neighboring cell

Cytotoxic T cell CD8+

Released perforins, granzymes, granulysin

Infected cell death

+ Complement components

Antibody-mediated cell cytotoxicity

Figure 13-4. Immune-mediated pathologic damage due to viral infection. Damage to tissue may be initiated by response to released viral antigens and to viral antigens presented by MHC molecules on the surface of infected host cells. Released antigens allow development of antibody responses (*left side*), leading to deposition on the surface of infected targets and cellular destruction by complement mediation. T_H cells release cytokines that assist cytotoxic lymphocytes to induce killing of target cells (*right side*). During both processes, bystander killing of surrounding tissue may occur, leading to manifestation of pathology.

IFN-α and IFN-β, secreted molecules that bind to specific receptors on adjacent cells to protect them against subsequent infection by progeny viruses. There are at least 17 different subtypes of IFN-α but only one subtype of IFN-β. In addition to direct antiviral effects, IFN-α and -β enhance expression of class I and class II MHC molecules on infected cells, in effect increasing viral antigen presentation to specific T_H and cytotoxic T cells. A functionally related molecule, IFN-γ, produced by T_H1 cells, cytotoxic lymphocytes, and NK cells, is a potent activator of macrophages and a powerful antiviral immunomodulating agent.

A more specific approach is to synthesize antibodies that bind to viral pathogens to mark them for attack and clearance by other elements of the immune system. Vaccination (immunoprophylaxis) induces a primed state so that secondary exposure to a pathogen generates a rapid immune response leading to accelerated elimination of the organism and protection against onset of clinical disease. Success

depends on the generation of memory T and B cells and the presence in the serum of antivirus-specific neutralizing antibody. Neutralizing antibodies work to inhibit viral attachment, penetration, uncoating, and even viral replication. Alternatively, non-neutralizing antibodies can be quite therapeutically functional, assisting in viral clearance by marking the virus for phagocytosis by monocytes. Antiviral vaccines are effective when presented to the host in a manner that is similar to natural exposure to viral antigens, thus generating protective immunity. This may be accomplished through active immunization with live modified viral strains, with inactivated virus particles, and with subunit vaccines (Table 13-2). In general, active immunization leads to long-lasting immunity. Alternatively, passive antiviral treatment is possible by administration of high-titer, specific antivirus antibodies (hyperimmune globulin) that confer host resistance. Passive administration leads to fast-acting but temporary immunity to imminent or ongoing exposure.

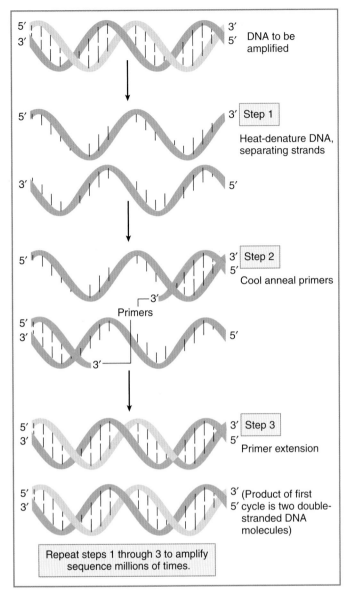

5′ / 3′ — DNA to be amplified

Step 1 — Heat-denature DNA, separating strands

Step 2 — Cool anneal primers

Primers

Step 3 — Primer extension

(Product of first cycle is two double-stranded DNA molecules)

Repeat steps 1 through 3 to amplify sequence millions of times.

Figure 13-5. Diagnostic evaluation of viral infection by PCR. Viral identification can be accomplished by multiple means, including cell culture, microscopic identification, serologic methods to detect antiviral antibodies, direct detection of viral antigens, or detection of nucleic acids by polymerase chain reaction (PCR). The method of PCR amplification of viral nucleic acids is depicted here.

KEY POINTS ABOUT THERAPY AND PROPHYLAXIS FOR VIRAL INFECTIONS

- Interferons are a natural part of the immediate protective host response, which is elicited upon invasion by viruses.

- Among the few successful chemotherapeutic agents that inhibit viral replication are nucleoside analogs that compete with normal nucleotides for incorporation into viral DNA or RNA and protease inhibitors that interfere with virus assembly.

- Immunization with subunit vaccines or live attenuated viruses increases both antibody production and long-term protective cell-mediated responses directed at viruses upon subsequent infection.

TABLE 13-2. Virus Vaccines

Vaccine Class	Virus	Comments
Live virus vaccines	Adenovirus Chickenpox Measles Mumps Poliovirus (Sabin vaccine) Rotavirus Rubella Smallpox (variola) Yellow fever	Active immunization using avirulent attenuated strains Effective at inducing antibodies and cytotoxic lymphocyte responses
Killed virus vaccines	Hepatitis A Influenza Poliovirus (Salk vaccine) Rabies	Active immunization using heat or chemically inactive virus particles Vaccination may be combined with other viruses (polyvalent)
Subunit vaccines	Adenovirus	Active immunization using purified proteins
Polypeptide vaccines	Hepatitis B	Active immunization using synthesized polypeptide protein sequences
DNA vaccines (evaluation only)	HIV Influenza	Experimental Useful for induction of cytotoxic T lymphocyte response
Passive antibodies	Hepatitis A Hepatitis B Measles Mumps Rabies Respiratory syncytial virus Rubella Varicella-zoster (VZV)	Injected purified antibodies obtained from another source Short-lived function with little value when given after disease onset

Clinical Virology

CONTENTS

Viruses are entities that infect and replicate within host cells, able to direct cellular machinery to synthesize new infectious particles. The extent of infection and associated pathology depends upon the number of virions infecting the host, as well as the physical damage and trauma associated with the infective process. Many times, host recognition of viral antigens and immune response contribute greatly to disease and pathologic manifestations. Selected viruses of clinical significance are listed in Table 14-1.

●●● RESPIRATORY VIRUSES

The main agents for clinical respiratory infections include the adenovirus, parainfluenza virus, respiratory syncytial virus (RSV), and rhinovirus. These viruses cause disease in the upper respiratory tract that leads to symptoms of pharyngitis (sore throat) with accompanying coryza (nasal discharge), tonsillitis, inflammation of the sinuses and middle ear, fever, and myalgia (muscle pain). Infection of the lower respiratory tract may induce bronchitis with inflammation of the larynx and trachea, exhausting cough and wheezing, and bronchopneumonia.

Adenovirus

The adenovirus group represents approximately 50 identified species of nonenveloped, double-stranded DNA viruses. The adenoviruses are frequently associated with asymptomatic respiratory tract infection that produces cellular cytolysis in the pharynx and subsequent host inflammation and cytokine response from immune T cells. Of interest, certain species easily lend themselves to genetic engineering and have the potential for gene therapy in clinical settings. During lytic infection, the adenovirus enters human epithelial cells, replicates, and causes host cell death. Transition to latent infection involves lymphoid tissue, where virus may remain dormant for longer periods of time. There are reports that adenovirus infection may be linked to oncogenesis and cancer, although this has not been firmly established. Clinical symptoms include acute respiratory disease and pharyngeal related fever; immunocompromised hosts are susceptible, and special care should be taken to monitor postoperative, therapeutically induced immunosuppression in transplant patients.

TABLE 14-1. Selected Viruses of Clinical Significance

Virus Class	Viral Agent	Clinical Manifestations
Respiratory virus	Parainfluenza Rhinovirus Severe acute respiratory syndrome (SARS) Respiratory syncytial virus (RSV)	Pharyngitis and coryza Tonsillitis and sinus inflammation Fever and myalgia
Childhood exanthem	Mumps Rubella virus and rubeola Erythema infectiosum Chickenpox	Exanthems Rash-like macules
Poxvirus	Smallpox Variola virus	Papulovesicular lesions
Enterovirus	Poliovirus Coxsackievirus	Meningitis Exanthems and myocarditis
Hepatitis virus	Hepatitis A–E	Liver dysfunction, hepatocellular carcinomas
Herpesvirus	HSV-1, HSV-2, CMV, EBV, VZV	Cold sores and fever blisters Mononucleosis Lymphomas
Rhabdovirus	Rabies virus *Lyssavirus*	Acute CNS infection
Papovavirus	Human papillomavirus (HPV)	Cutaneous or mucosal lesions
Retrovirus	HIV-1 and HIV-2 HTLV	AIDS, leukemia
Arbovirus	Dengue virus Yellow fever virus Japanese encephalitis virus West Nile virus	Viral hemorrhagic fever Encephalitis and meningitis
Prion	Prions	Spongiform encephalopathy
Emerging viral agent	Ebola virus *Hantavirus*	Hemorrhagic fever Pulmonary distress

Parainfluenza Virus

Parainfluenza viruses are paramyxoviruses that are the causative agents of nearly 40% of acute respiratory infections in infants and children. Human parainfluenzas are serotyped as paramyxoviruses 1 through 4; serotype 4 consists of subtypes A and B. The virus is acquired through inhalation of infected respiratory droplets, with the nasopharynx as the primary site of infection. The virus attaches to cell membranes by way of a hemagglutinin trimeric protein that binds cell surface glycoproteins with neuraminic acid residues. Clinical symptoms range from the simple common cold to croup, bronchitis, and bronchopneumonia. Symptoms are usually accompanied by a hoarse or "barking" cough, sometimes with a swollen epiglottis.

Rhinovirus

Rhinoviruses (among other viruses that infect the upper respiratory tract) cause the "common cold" or cold-like symptoms (discharging or blocked nasal passages, sneezing and rhinorrhea, and sore throat). There are greater than 120 serotypes, which are primarily spread by aerosolization. The most common route of infection is the nose, and infections do not spread to the lower respiratory or intestinal tracts. Infection spread is limited by simple washing of hands. Most rhinoviruses replicate in epithelial cells of the nasal mucosa, eventually leading to edema of connective tissue. Cellular destruction is commonly caused by immune response to viral infection and antigens and not by direct viral cytotoxic activity.

Coronavirus

Coronaviridae are best known as the second most frequent cause of the common cold. Although coronaviruses are known to cause disease in birds and pigs, recent studies indicate that the agent responsible for the severe acute respiratory syndrome (SARS) belongs to this genus. SARS is a serious, life-threatening viral infection that is thought to have mutated to a human transmissible form. The mortality rate of SARS is high compared with other common respiratory viral infections, with up to 10% of fatalities due to respiratory failure following symptoms of hypoxia, cough, and dyspnea (labored breathing).

Respiratory Syncytial Virus

Respiratory syncytial virus (RSV), a paramyxovirus, is the main cause of bronchiolitis (inflammation of the bronchioles) and pneumonia in children. As the name implies, infection in tissue culture causes cells to form syncytia, resulting in large, multinucleated cells.

●●● MUMPS, MEASLES, AND OTHER CHILDHOOD EXANTHEMS

Childhood viral-related exanthems (eruptive disease) include rubeola (measles) and rubella (German measles), chickenpox, roseola infantum, erythema infectiosum (a parvovirus; also called fifth disease). All these infections affect the respiratory system and are highly contagious. Unless immunocompromised, children with these illnesses recover fully without treatment. As with all viral infections, a heavy load may result in more severe complications, including pneumonia, heart and kidney damage, and encephalitis. In the United States and most of Europe, successful vaccination programs have limited the incidence of disease, although these viruses remain a major cause of childhood deaths in other regions of the globe. The MMR vaccine protects against measles, mumps, and rubella using live, attenuated viral antigens.

Mumps

Mumps is a paramyxovirus that causes inflammation of the salivary, parotid, and submaxillary glands. In adults, orchitis and oophoritis (inflammation of the testis and ovaries) may occur. A common clinical association is that of aseptic meningitis due to disseminated infection after viral crossing of the blood-brain barrier.

Rubella

Rubella virus, which causes German measles, is the single member of the *Rubivirus* genus of the togavirus family. Infection results in rash-like macules on the face, body, and limbs. There is associated lymphadenopathy at the back of the head and neck, which may proceed to arthralgia (joint pain) and symptoms of arthritis as infection disseminates. Special care should be taken regarding rubella infections of women during the first trimester of pregnancy, since spread of infection to the fetus will lead to congenital abnormalities (e.g., heart defects, deafness, and mental retardation) in the majority of cases.

Rubeola

Rubeola (measles) is a common childhood illness caused by a Morbillivirus, resulting in manifestation of a diagnostically distinst exanthema. The virus is spread through direct contact with nasal or throat discharge from an infected individual. The disease is very contagious and typically persists for one week to 10 days. The hallmark of infection is a rash that usually begins on the face and spreads to the rest of the host's body; infection is accompanied by fever and cough. After symptoms disappear, one is left with a lifelong immunity against subsequent infection.

Parvovirus

Erythema infectiosum caused by parvovirus B19 is similar to measles. It is also called fifth disease or "slapped cheek disease" because of its tropism for immature red cells (erythrotropism). This leads to the characteristic facial sequela of a lacy, pink, macular rash on the cheeks. Because of its predilection for immature RBCs, transmission from mother to fetus can be life-threatening for the unborn child.

Varicella

The causative agent for chickenpox (varicella) is a member of the human herpesvirus family. Infection occurs by inhalation with replication of the virus in the mucosa of the upper respiratory tract, followed by dissemination throughout regional lymph nodes. In the case of chickenpox, resulting pathology manifests as a macule that develops to a pustular lesion, which eventually crusts over. The virus has the ability to establish latent infection in neurons that can reactivate when cellular immunity is impaired or wanes due to advanced age. Varicella-zoster virus causes herpes zoster (shingles), a herpetic neuropathology in which reactivated virus travels through axons to infect the dermatome supplied by the sensory ganglion, thus introducing painful vesicular lesions on the skin. Another related herpesvirus, HHV6, is responsible for roseola infantum, causing a febrile illness with a rash in newborns.

●●● POXVIRUSES

Smallpox (variola) is an orthopox virus that has been virtually eliminated in humans as a result of international efforts to control disease through intense vaccination with cross-reactive vaccinia. Related pathogenic poxviruses in humans include those caused by cowpox and molluscum contagiosum, all of which cause papulovesicular lesions on the hands, forearms, or face. Monkeypox is a generalized infection that may be more invasive and involve lung tissue.

●●● ENTEROVIRUSES

Enteroviruses are members of the picornavirus family. They are orally or fecally transmissible; ingested viruses infect cells of the oral cavity and pharyngeal mucosa, as well as draining lymphoid tissue (tonsil, cervical, and eventually mesenteric). After replication, they are shed into the alimentary tract and intestinal tissue. The enteroviruses include poliovirus, coxsackieviruses A and B, echovirus, and hepatitis A. The overall clinical symptoms are typically mild but may on occasion cause serious persistent disease with continued shedding of virions for months to years.

Poliovirus

Prior to the introduction of vaccines, paralytic poliomyelitis was a major health threat. Introduction of the Salk vaccine, using inactivated virions, and the Sabin vaccine, using attenuated virions, quickly led to high levels of protection in the general population. There are three serotypes of poliovirus (1, 2, and 3) with serotype 1 being the most prevalent. Infection with poliovirus can be life-threatening; within 1 week after infection the virus has the potential to disseminate, entering the blood supply and spreading to the anterior horn of the spinal cord and then to the motor cortex of the brain. Paralysis ensues, dependent upon which neurons are infected and the amount of damage caused during infection.

Coxsackievirus

Coxsackievirus types A and B can cause pathogenic infection. Coxsackie type A is typically associated with exanthems, while both types A and B can lead to myocarditis. If untreated, infection may result in an aseptic meningitis involving headache and fever, stiff neck, and malaise. Coxsackie type A can cause painful mouth ulcers of the tongue and hand-foot-and-mouth disease, exhibited by blisters on the hands and feet. It may also cause Bornholm disease (sometimes called the devil's grip), manifested as sharp chest/side pains (epidemic pleurodynia).

Echoviruses

Echoviruses (*enteric cytopathic human orphan* viruses) cause symptoms similar to rhinovirus infection. They also may cause exanthems and myocarditis, similarly to the coxsackieviruses described. Rashes may be maculopapular, similar to rubella (German measles), or of a lighter, subcutaneous form (roseola-like, vesicular, or petechial).

●●● HEPATITIS VIRUSES

Five recognized hepatitis viruses are known to cause liver-related pathology. They are hepatitis A, B, C, D, and E. Hepatitis A and E are enterically transmitted, while the others are parenterally spread (Fig. 14-1). Hepatitis A (called infectious hepatitis) is caused by the picornavirus enterovirus 72; hepatitis E is a calicivirus. In both cases, the virus is spread by fecal-oral route, it replicates in the intestinal tract prior to infecting hepatocytes, and it eventually is spread through the stool.

Human hepatitis B (HBV) is a hepadnavirus, similar to strains found in the woodchuck and duck. The virus is spread by needles, sexual encounter, and from mother to fetus during birth. HBV replicates in the liver, with a large load of virus particles shed during infection that are available for immune recognition; antibodies to the surface antigen (HBsAg) are a useful diagnostic tool for infection detection. Persistent infection leads to chronic liver damage with accompanying cirrhosis and potential for development of hepatocellular carcinoma. Hepatitis C is a flavivirus that also causes hepatocellular carcinomas. Hepatitis D, or "delta agent," is a defective virus that requires HBV to replicate, and it seems to exacerbate symptoms related to HBV. Finally, a related hepatitis G flavivirus has been identified but does not seem to be a major cause of liver disease.

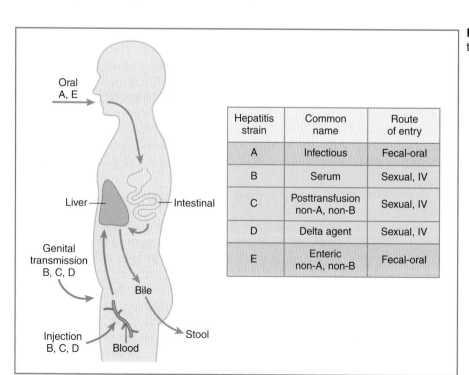

Hepatitis strain	Common name	Route of entry
A	Infectious	Fecal-oral
B	Serum	Sexual, IV
C	Posttransfusion non-A, non-B	Sexual, IV
D	Delta agent	Sexual, IV
E	Enteric non-A, non-B	Fecal-oral

Figure 14-1. Routes of transmission for the hepatitis viruses.

TABLE 14-2. Properties of Human Herpesviruses

Virus Strain	Common Name	Clinical Manifestation	Features
Human herpes simplex virus 1	HHSV1, HSV-1	Cold sores, or fever blisters (oral, keratitis)	Cytopathic progression to latent infection of neurons and ganglia
Human herpes simplex virus 2	HHSV2, HSV-2	Painful genital blisters	Similar to HHSV1
Human cytomegalovirus	HCMV	Fever and lymphocytoses	Mononucleosis-like illness
Epstein-Barr virus	EBV	Lymphadenopathy, sore throat, hepatosplenomegaly	Persistent in B lymphocytes (Burkitt's lymphoma)
Varicella-zoster virus	VZV	Chickenpox and shingles	Latent infection in neurons
Human herpesvirus 6	HHV6	Roseola infantum	T-cell lymphotropic virus
Human herpesvirus 7	HHSV7, HHV7	No known diseases	"Orphan" virus
Human herpesvirus 8	HHSV8, HHV8	Primary effusion lymphoma	Considered agent responsible for Kaposi sarcoma and Castleman disease

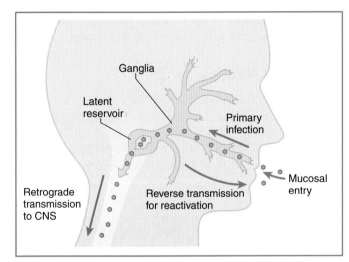

Figure 14-2. Primary herpesvirus infection and reactivation of latent infection. Herpes simplex virus establishes a primary infection of the skin or oral mucosa and spreads to nearby ganglia, where it may remain latent. Upon reactivation, reverse travel of virus in a ganglion allows spread to skin or mucosa, causing occurrence of surface lesions. Retrograde transmission may occur as well, leading to meningitis upon infection of the CNS.

NEUROSCIENCE

Efferent Motoneurons

Somatic efferent motoneurons originate in the spinal cord and synapse with muscle fibers to direct contraction of skeletal muscle. These motoneurons are asymmetric units composed of a dendrite, a soma, and axons, which may be several feet in length. These neurons may be exploited by viruses (such as herpes or varicella) where retrograde transmission allows axonal transport of infectious agent to other regions of the body.

with cytopathic infections that progress to latent infection of neurons and ganglia (Fig. 14-2). In many cases, reactivation occurs under conditions of stress and immunosuppression, or even unrelated immune hypersensitivity reactions. Pathology of vesicular lesions occurs via both direct cytolytic activity and immune response attacking infected tissue. Common manifestations include cold sores, or fever blisters, which may often be seen around the mouth and lips. Of interest, almost all adults have been exposed to HHSV1 at some time, with positive antibody titers present in serum. HHSV2 is the causative agent for genital herpes.

Cytomegalovirus

Human cytomegalovirus (HCMV) infects most individuals within the first few years of childhood, with approximately 70% of adults having IgG antibodies specific for cytomegalovirus antigens. The virus is harbored in CD4+ and CD8+ cell phenotypes. Virus is secreted in saliva; infection may result in a mononucleosis-like illness associated with hepatitis, fever, and lymphocytoses (increase in blood lymphocytes). Infection of healthy individuals does not lead to symptoms; however, transplant patients and immunosuppressed individuals are at much greater risk for development of infection-related pathologies.

●●● HERPESVIRUSES

The herpesviruses include eight members that cause pathology, including the varicella-zoster virus and HHV6 described above. In all cases, latent infection is established after a primary persistent and lytic indication, sometimes lying dormant throughout the lifetime of an individual. Table 14-2 lists properties of the herpesviruses.

HHSV1 and HHSV2

Human herpes simplex virus types 1 and 2 (HHSV1 and HHSV2) are characterized by infectious virions that begin

Burkitt's Lymphoma

Burkitt's lymphoma is a high-grade B-cell lymphoma associated with EBV. The basis of the pathology is thought to occur through infection and transformation of B cells leading to malignancy through chromosomal translocation events. The most common translocation moves the protooncogene *Myc*-containing segment of chromosome 8 to chromosome 14q band 32, placing it close to the immunoglobulin heavy chain gene and resulting in Myc overexpression.

Epstein-Barr Virus (EBV)

Epstein-Barr virus is similar to HCMV in that nearly all adults have antibodies specific for EBV antigens. The virus is persistent in B lymphocytes and is the agent responsible for infectious mononucleosis and X-linked lymphoproliferative syndrome. Infectious mononucleosis ("kissing disease") is characterized by lymphadenopathy, sore throat, and hepatosplenomegaly; because of the predilection of B cells for infection, atypical lymphocytes are present in peripheral blood. When reactivated, EBV can cause Burkitt's lymphoma and other carcinomas.

HHSV7 and HHSV8

Human herpesvirus 7 is an "orphan" virus that has been identified and isolated, but no known diseases have been attributed to HHSV7. Human herpesvirus 8 (HHSV8) is thought to be the agent responsible for the Kaposi sarcoma that is characteristic of later stage HIV infection.

●●● RHABDOVIRUSES

Lyssavirus

Lyssaviruses are rhabdoviruses. The genus *Lyssavirus* includes the neurotropic rabies virus, the Mokola virus, the Duvenhage virus, and the European and Australian bat lyssaviruses. The classic madness associated with rabies virus is well documented through history and popular literature. Dogs serve as a reservoir for disease, as do coyotes, wolves, jackals,

skunks, raccoons, and foxes. Shortly after infection, the virus migrates through peripheral nerves and enters the brain, causing acute pathology within the central nervous system (CNS), leading to neurologic disorders and sometimes death.

●●● PAPOVAVIRUSES

Papillomaviruses

Human papillomaviruses (HPVs) are papovaviruses that are clinically defined according to their ability to induce cutaneous or mucosal lesions (Table 14-3). Mechanistically, these viruses infect basal epidermal keratinocytes, where they lay dormant until epidermal cells migrate to the skin surface. This induces the virus to replicate, altering the appearance of host tissue and resulting in cutaneous or mucosal localized verrucae (warts), which appear as hyperkeratotic nodules. Papillomaviruses have anatomic preferences, some causing lesions on the skin surface while others cause genital or anal lesions. In addition, there is strong evidence that certain papillomaviruses are linked to cervical and genital cancers.

JC and BK Viruses

Two additional members of the papovavirus family are known to infect humans. The JC virus replicates in neural tissue and is associated with progressive, multifocal leukocyte encephalopathy. The BK virus has been isolated from the urinary tract, indicative of the kidney being the site of infec-

TABLE 14-3. Papillomavirus Infections

Cutaneous Papilloma	Anatomic Site
Common wart (verruca vulgaris)	Hands
Plantar wart	Feet
Butcher's wart	Hand
Flat wart	Arms, face, knees
Extragenital Bowen's disease	Extremities, head
Epidermodysplasia verruciformis	Exposed skin
Mucosal papilloma	Mucosa
Laryngeal	Larynx
Conjunctival	Arms, face, knees
Oral	Mouth
Anogenital papilloma	Genital, anal areas
Condyloma acuminatum	Genital, anal areas
Cervical intraepithelial neoplasia	Neck
Bowen's disease	Groin
Buschke-Löwenstein tumor	Glans penis, perianal area
Vulvar intraepithelial neoplasia	Genital area
Penile/anal intraepithelial neoplasia	Genital area

Keratinized Epidermal Layers of the Skin

An outer protective layer of keratinized stratified squamous epithelium covers the dermis. Keratinocytes primarily within the stratum lucidum and stratum corneum produce a fibrous scleroprotein that is the chief structural component of hair and nails.

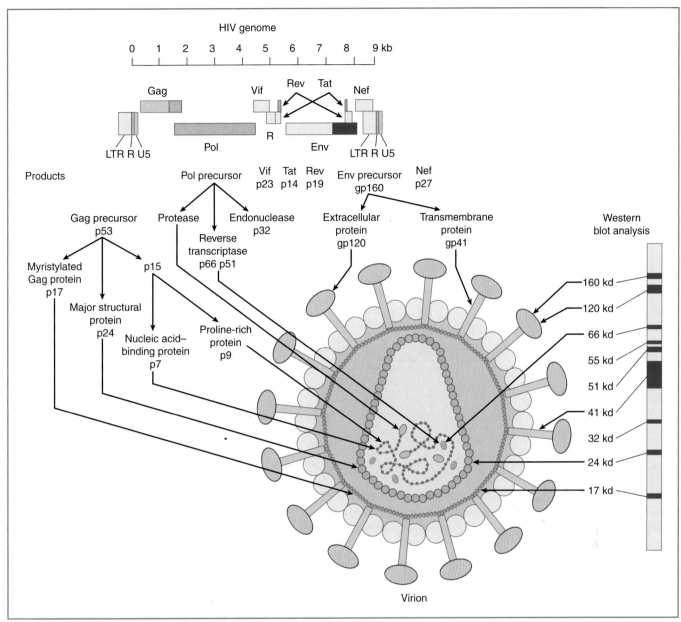

Figure 14-3. Structure of HIV. The HIV retrovirus comprises an outer envelope glycoprotein coat surrounding a lipid bilayer. Internal group antigens provide core protein and scaffold structure. Internal reverse transcriptase and regulatory proteins interact with viral RNA, allowing virus gene expression and protein assembly for replicating virions.

tion. BK virus may cause interstitial nephritis and cystitis. Neither causes major pathologic damage unless the patient is immunocompromised or immunosuppressed.

●●● RETROVIRUSES

Retroviruses require reverse transcription of their single-stranded RNA genome to a double-stranded DNA intermediate for integration into the host cell genome. The retroviruses represent infectious agents that may be oncogenic or cytolytic. This group includes the slow-acting lentiviruses of which AIDS-associated HIV-1 and HIV-2 are members, having high clinical importance and enormous social and economic impact throughout the world.

Human Immunodeficiency Virus (HIV)

The human immunodeficiency virus–1 (HIV-1) is the retrovirus most commonly associated with HIV infection in the United States and Europe. HIV-2, which has high nucleotide sequence homology to HIV-1, is prevalent in regions of Africa. Both are lentiviruses that infect CD4+ cells, including T helper lymphocytes, macrophages, and other cell types. The gp120 virus surface antigen binds with high affinity to the cell surface CD4, promoting fusion between virus and cell membranes. Coreceptor chemokine receptors CXCR4 and CCR5 may also play a role in internalization, as well as immunoglobulins that assist in antibody-dependent uptake (Fig. 14-3). The natural history of HIV depicts the outcome of

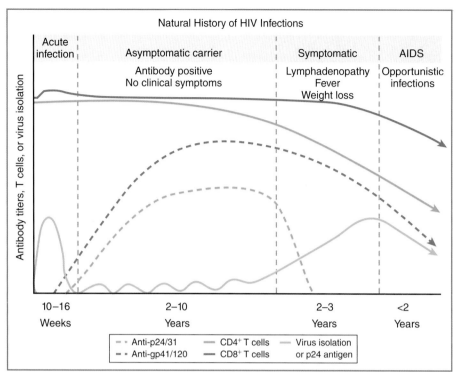

Figure 14-4. Natural history of HIV. Infection of CD4+ lymphocytes (and other cell types) leads to virus production and cytolysis or long-term latent infection that progresses from primary infection through late symptomatic infection (AIDS). Accompanying this process are profound defects in T_H and cytotoxic cell activity, with concomitant development of opportunistic infections.

HIV infection, which leads to destruction of lymphocytes and development of AIDS (Fig. 14-4).

Human T Lymphocyte Virus (HTLV)

The human T lymphocyte virus is an oncogenic retrovirus transmitted by human contact, associated with adult T-cell leukemia. The different subtypes of HTLV are classified according to their ability to infect T lymphocytes. Presentation of infection may be asymptomatic, give rise to neurologic disorders, or result in lymphoproliferative events. HTLV-l infection is the main type associated with acute adult T-cell leukemia.

●●● ARBOVIRUSES

Arboviruses are primarily transmitted by arthropod vectors, including those viruses spread by mosquitos and ticks. The virus has a reservoir in another species (zoonotic), with humans being a secondary host for the infective agent.

Dengue Virus

Dengue virus is a flavivirus, which has four related subtypes. The virus is spread by a bite of the mosquito *Aedes aegypti* or *Aedes albopictus*. The major pathology during infection is due to increased capillary permeability, which leads to subsequent pleural effusion, ascites, and thrombocytopenia. Petechial skin hemorrhages may occur, as well as gastrointestinal bleeding.

Yellow Fever

Yellow fever is another flavivirus that causes viral hemorrhagic fever. It is commonly found in Africa and South America and is spread by multiple mosquito species. The disease may lead to liver failure, renal insufficiency, and in some cases proteinuria (excess protein in urine). The jaundice associated with the disease led to its common name.

Japanese Encephalitis Virus

Japanese encephalitis virus is a mosquito-borne (*Culex tritaeniorhychnus*) flavivirus found in East and Southeast Asia. Domestic pigs and wild birds serve as reservoirs. The disease manifests as acute encephalitis, with rigor, including neck stiffness, muscular weakness, and partial paralysis, and cachexia (wasting).

West Nile Virus

West Nile virus causes a viral-induced encephalitis and meningitis. The virus is endemic in the Near East, Africa, and Southwest Asia; recently it has been found in North America. Wild birds transmit the virus by way of multiple mosquito species (*Culex, Aedes,* and *Anopheles*). The virus crosses the blood-brain barrier and infects brain parenchyma and the leptomeninges.

Tick-Borne Encephalitis

Tick-borne encephalitis is yet another flavivirus that causes disease involving the CNS. The disease manifests as menin-

TABLE 14-4. Some Emerging Viral Pathogens

Viral Agent	Family	Infection	Zoonotic Reservoir
Ebola virus	Filoviridae	Hemorrhagic fever	Possibly primates
Marburg virus	Filoviridae	Hemorrhagic fever	Possibly African green monkey
Lassa virus	Arenaviridae	Hemorrhagic fever	Rodents
African swine fever virus	Iridoviridae (formerly)		Warthog + tick vector
Morbillivirus, equine (Nipah virus)	Paramyxoviridae	Encephalitis, respiratory disease	Horse
Hantavirus	Bunyaviridae	Pulmonary distress	Rodents
Lyssavirus, bat	Rhabdoviridae	Rabies-like illness	Bat
Severe acute respiratory syndrome (SARS)	Coronaviridae	Pulmonary distress	Birds

gitis, encephalitis, or meningoencephalitis. The reservoir is the *Ixodes* tick, and the disease is found in Russia and East Asia.

Vesiculovirus

The vesicular stomatitis virus (VSV) is also a rhabdovirus. It is thought that infection may be transmitted by sandflies and mosquitoes, with humans infected directly by the transcutaneous route.

Other Arboviruses

Ross River virus is an alphavirus in the togavirus family. It is transmitted via mosquitos and causes polyarthritis and acute fever, with the majority of cases reported in Australia and the South Pacific islands. Rift valley fever is also spread by mosquitos and is caused by *Phlebovirus* of the Bunyaviridae family.

●●● PRIONS

Prion disease is a form of spongiform encephalopathy thought to be of viral origin. The etiology is related to a prion protein that has the same primary amino acid sequence as a host protein found at low levels in healthy brain tissue. The prion protein has an abnormal conformation and triggers conversion of the normal host cellular isoform to an infectious form. Accumulations of the abnormal form are deposited as amyloid within the brain. The diseases associated with this infection are Creutzfeldt-Jakob disease, Gerstmann-Sträussler-Scheinker disease, and kuru.

●●● EMERGING VIRAL PATHOGENS

Emerging viral pathogens are viruses that suddenly appear in the environment with severe economic and social impact. These agents are usually extremely virulent and often are originally zoonotic. The species-jumping infectious agent finds a suitable host in humans, either through mutation or adaptation. A list of emerging viral pathogens is given in Table 14-4.

Mycology

15

●●● BASIC MYCOLOGY

Fungi are filamentous, spore-producing, eukaryotic organisms that do not contain chlorophyll. There are more than 100,000 species that grow as saprophytes (requiring organic material for energy), with beneficial use in production of foods such as cheese, wine, and beer. However, nearly 300 species are pathogenic for man. Mycotic species are known to cause allergic reactions (to molds and spores), elicit toxic effects (mycotoxicosis) upon ingestion of fungal products, and lead to infection with severity determined by the immune status of the host.

Fungal Structure and Classification

The mycotic species include molds, yeasts, and higher fungi. The phyla of medically important fungi are listed in Table 15-1. Fungi have a complex structural cell wall made primarily of the polysaccharides chitin, glucans, and mannans. The membrane is bilayered with inclusion of sterol components (ergosterol and zymosterol), in contrast to the cholesterol typically found in higher eukaryotic membranes. Fungi are usually aerobic and exhibit both sexual and asexual forms of reproduction.

Almost all fungi form filaments called *hyphae,* which are the filamentous subunits of molds and mushrooms. They may exist as septate forms (with cross-walls) or as aseptate coenocytic forms (without cross-walls). A colony or mass of multibranched intertwined hyphae is referred to as a *mycelium*; a fungal body may also be called a *thallus.* Yeasts are single-celled forms of fungi that generally reproduce by budding. Under differing environmental conditions, dimorphic fungi can change morphology between yeast and hyphal structures. Some fungi produce spores, formed asexually or sexually, which may contribute to allergic responses in certain individuals. Others reproduce through fragmentation. The different forms are depicted in Figure 15-1.

Fungal Pathogenesis

Fungi do not produce endotoxins or exotoxins. Rather, infection in many cases is due to colonization of the organism at local or systemic tissue sites. Low pH, fatty acids, and rapid turnover of skin surface epithelial cell layers limit infections. Antibodies (primarily IgA with some assistance by IgG) at mucosal surfaces may also contribute by limiting growth and spread of fungal agents.

Agents may be classified according to tissue colonized. Superficial mycoses are limited to the skin and hair. For example, tinea nigra and tinea versicolor are superficial skin infections giving rise to macular lesions. Black piedra and white piedra colonize hair shafts, resulting in brittle hair. Cutaneous mycoses include infections of keratinized tissue, usually hair and nails. Dermatophytes, such as those causing ringworm of the scalp (tinea capitis), folliculitis (tinea barbae), and athlete's foot (tinea pedis) are included in this category. Subcutaneous mycoses, usually introduced by trauma or breach of dermal tissue, involve infections of subcutaneous fascia, muscle, and deeper epidermal layers. Chromomycosis caused by soil fungi results in abscesses and lesion development along lymphatics as infection spreads. Mycetomas and sporotrichosis infection may also cause cutaneous lesions represented as pustule nodules as organisms are cleared from subcutaneous sites. All three (superficial, subcutaneous, and cutaneous mycoses) are typically non-invasive infections. Systemic mycoses on the other hand can be life-threatening, especially when the host is immuno-compromised. While normal immune responses leave the host asymptomatic, opportunistic disease may ensue if an individual is immunosuppressed. Systemic infections result from inhalation of pathogenic fungal spores, followed by differen-tiation and dissemination to other tissue sites. Histoplasmo-sis, coccidiomycosis, and blastomycosis are three dimorphic fungi present as mold forms in soil and yeast in tissue.

TABLE 15-1. Phyla of Medically Important Fungi

Phyla	Spore Type	Characteristics	Reproduction
Ascomycota	Ascospores	Penicillium mold, yeast, *Aspergillus* aflatoxin	Sexual reproduction in a sac called an ascus
Deuteromycetes (mitosporic fungi)	Imperfect fungus	Ringworm, athlete's foot	No formation of sexual spores
Oomycetes	Zoospores	Aquatic "water molds"	Asexual spore reproduction
Zygomycota	Zygospores, sporangiospores	Bread molds, rice fermenters	Sexual reproduction by gametes as well as asexual reproduction
Basidiomycota	Basidiospores	Causative agents of plant diseases	Sexual reproduction in a sac called a basidium

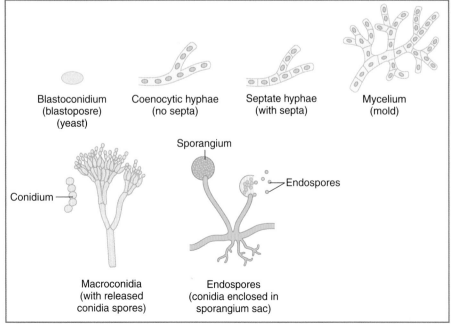

Blastoconidium (blastoposre) (yeast)

Coenocytic hyphae (no septa)

Septate hyphae (with septa)

Mycelium (mold)

Sporangium

Conidium

Endospores

Macroconidia (with released conidia spores)

Endospores (conidia enclosed in sporangium sac)

Figure 15-1. Fungal morphology. The growth of fungi generally involves two phases: vegetative and reproductive. In the vegetative phase, the cells are haploid and divide mitotically. Most fungi exist as molds with hyphae, but some fungi exist as unicellular yeast cells. Some fungi can change their morphology and are termed dimorphic. In the reproductive phase, fungi undergo either asexual or sexual reproduction. Asexual reproduction involves the generation of spores.

Although usually self-limiting, dissemination to other tissue sites may occur, with ensuing destructive lesion development.

Mycotoxicoses are caused by ingestion of fungal toxins in contaminated foods. Ergotism, caused by ergot alkaloids from *Claviceps purpurea* released into grains, leads to pronounced vascular and neurologic disorders due to inhibition of epinephrine. These alkaloids include lysergic acid diethylamide (LSD), a psychotropic agent. Additional psychotropic toxins include those released from *Psilocybe*. Ingestion of *Amanita* mushrooms and associated amanitine and phalloidin toxins can lead to liver damage. *Aspergillus flavus* aflatoxins, found in contaminated grains and peanuts, are bisfuranocoumarin metabolites (coumarin derivatives) that cause hepatic hemorrhage and sever liver damage.

Allergic reactions to fungal spores are dependent upon the host's susceptibility, combining deleterious hypersensitive and antibody (IgE)–mediated responses. In many cases, immediate asthmatic reactions occur, with associated bronchoconstriction due to antibody-mediated release of histamines from mast cells and eosinophils.

Antifungal Agents

Because the cell wall consists primarily of chitin, fungal agents are not susceptible to common antibiotics that inhibit peptidoglycan synthesis. Effective therapy employs a combi-

nation of proper delivery to the site of infection (superficial vs. systemic) and directed activity against fungus-specific targets. For example, superficial infection of the skin or hair may be treated by site-specific cleansing in combination with topical applications. Subcutaneous or systemic infections require more aggressive and prolonged treatment. Targets against membrane sterols are particularly effective (nystatin, amphotericin B), as are azole derivatives that inhibit ergosterol biosynthesis (miconazole, fluconazole, ketoconazole). Grisans (griseofulvin) may be given orally to treat more invasive dermatophytes, working to inhibit microtubular function (Fig. 15-2).

Laboratory Diagnosis of Fungal Infections

Superficial and cutaneous mycoses may be identified by microscopic analysis, either by analysis of wet skin scrapings or visualization after staining. For visualization, treatment of skin with alkaline solution dissolves tissue, leaving resistant material available for further staining and identification by morphologic analysis. Identification by culture is possible, but because of the ubiquitous nature of fungal entities, the laboratory procedures must take into account the possibility of airborne contamination. For culture procedures, slow-growing organisms are cultured on Sabouraud's agar, which typically contains high levels of antibiotics to inhibit bacterial growth. More recent methods of identification include PCR analysis for specific DNA sequences and ELISA analysis to confirm fungal antigens. Diagnosis of dermatophytes requires recovery of organisms from lesions. Systemic mycoses are usually identified serologically and immunologically, with confirmation by culture and PCR performed on material isolated from infected tissue.

Immune Response to Fungal Agents

The major immune responses to fungal agents are delayed-type hypersensitivity and granulomatous responses (Fig. 15-3). However, not much is known about immune response to fungal agents; rather disease and pathology more often than not ensue when there is a failure in one arm of immunity. Cellular immunity appears to be the most important immunologic factor in resistance to fungal infections, although humoral responses (antibodies) may play a role. The importance of cellular reactions is indicated by the intense mononuclear infiltrate and granulomatous reactions that occur in tissues infected with fungi and by the fact that fungal infections are frequently associated with depressed immune reactivity of the delayed type (opportunistic infections). Chronic mucocutaneous candidiasis refers to persistent or recurrent infection by *Candida albicans* of mucous membranes, nails, and skin. Patients with this disease generally have a form of immune deviation (i.e., a depression of cellular immune reactions), with high levels of humoral antibody. Fungi appear to be resistant to the effects of antibody, so that cell-mediated immunity (CMI) is needed for effective resistance.

Figure 15-2. Molecular structure of selected antifungal agents.

Amphotericin B

Ketoconazole

Griseofulvin

Figure 15-3. Immune response to fungal agents. Gross pathology of lung tissue demonstrates fungus-induced granulomatous pneumonitis (**A**) and associated PAS-stained *Histoplasma* located within giant cells on histologic examination (**B**). Similar cellular response is evident upon infection with *Aspergillus* (**C**) shown with silver stain, caused by antigens released from the etiologic agent isolated from sinus maxillary tissue (**D**). (Part A reprinted with permission from Buja LM, Netter FH, Krueger GRF: *Netter's Illustrated Human Pathology*. Philadelphia: Elsevier, 2004.)

●●● CLINICAL MYCOLOGY

Superficial and Cutaneous Mycoses

The superficial mycoses include those that superficially infect skin or hair (Fig. 15-4). *Malassezia furfur* (tinea versicolor, pityriasis versicolor) infection of the skin causes hypo- or hyperpigmented macular lesions along the trunk of the body. *Exophiala werneckii* (tinea nigra) infection is usually asymptomatic and superficial, with hypopigmented areas appearing on the palms or on tanned skin. Associated lesions are usually flat and dark, owing to infection of stratum corneum layers of the epidermis. Piedra is a general term for fungal infection of hair shafts. *Piedraia hortae* (black piedra) infection results in hard black deposits along the hair shafts, while *Trichosporon beigelii* (white piedra) forms white deposits similar to a collar-like sleeve around hair follicles.

Cutaneous mycoses of the skin, hair, or nails are caused by dermatophytes belonging to three genera: *Epidermophyton*, *Microsporum*, and *Trichophyton*. Some instances may also be defined by *Candida* (yeast) infection. *Trichophyton rubrum*, *Trichophyton mentagrophytes*, and *Epidermophyton floccosum* are causative agents of athlete's foot, resulting in chronic scaly tinea pedis (scales on soles and heels). These same agents, along with *Candida* may also cause acute infection of the groin (tinea cruris, jock itch), often accompanied by athlete's foot. Although less common, these same agents, along with *Microsporum canis*, may infect skinfolds of the anus (tinea corporis), leading to annular lesions that are pustulous. *Trichophyton verrucosum* is the agent implicated in folliculitis of the facial hair (tinea barbae).

Ringworm of the scalp skin and hair (tinea capitis) is also considered a cutaneous mycosis, characterized as anthropophilic (epidemic, *Microsporum audouinii*) or zoophilic (nonepidemic, *Microsporum canis* or *Trichophyton mentagrophytes*). Anthropophilic tinea capitis is characterized by noninflammatory, grayish patches of hair and may be spread by contact with infected headgear. Zoophilic tinea capitis is typically of greater inflammatory nature, with resulting baldness (alopecia). *Trichophyton tonsurans* tinea capitis is very common in children and causes infections within the hair (endothrix). *Trichophyton schoenleinii* (tinea favus) is a more aggressive disease, with scalp scarring and hair loss occurring if not treated in a timely manner.

Candida spp (discussed below) are normal fungal flora inhabitants of the intestines. However, it should be noted that some species, such as *Candida albicans*, may cause dermatomycoses and ensuing skin lesions (e.g., vulvovaginitis), or otomycosis (infection of the auditory canal) and onychomycosis (infection of the fingernails). Thrush, infection of the tongue and inner mouth, is prevalent in immunocompromised individuals, especially those with late-stage HIV infection.

Three genera of actinomycetes were thought to be fungi but have more recently been shown to be bacteria that are related to mycobacteria. Two of these are discussed in Chapter 12: *Actinomyces* and acid-fast *Nocardia*. The third group, *Streptomyces*, causes a subcutaneous disease known

Figure 15-4. Locations of superficial and cutaneous mycoses.

Cerebral chromomycosis: *Hormodendrum; Phialophora*

Rhinospridiosis: *Rhinosproidium*

Tinea barbae (folliculitis): *Trichophyton*

Lymphocutaneous sporotrichosis: *Sporothrix*

Tinea versicolor (trunk), Pityriasis versicolor: *Malassezia*

Tinea corporis (anus): *Microsporum*

Eumycetoma (fascia and bones): *Pseudallescheria; Madurella*

White/black piedra (scalp, body, genital area): *Trichosporon; Piedraia*

Cutaneous mycoses (skin, hair, nails): *Epidermophyton, Microsporum, Trichophyton, Candida*

Exophiala werneckii (tinea nigra)

as fungus tumor (mycetoma), which if untreated can penetrate deep into tissue and infect bone material. The streptomycetes are aerobic like *Nocardia*.

Subcutaneous Mycoses

Three common subcutaneous mycoses are those causing sporotrichosis, chromomycosis, and mycetoma. All represent disease caused by saprophytic (soil-growing) fungi that enter tissue, usually through trauma. *Sporothrix schenckii* is the causative agent of lymphocutaneous sporotrichosis and is the most common form of subcutaneous nodular fungal disease. Clinical presentation demonstrates lesions following lymphatic vessels, with ulceration. Although lesions may be chronic, there is only minimal instance of systemic spread. Chromomycosis (or chromoblastomycosis) caused by dematiaceous (black-brown) fungi can appear as subcutaneous lesions that manifest along lymphatics. In many cases, such as seen in verrucous dermatitis, granulomatous response ensues, leading to histologic presence of giant cells and lymphocytes in infected tissue. Cerebral chromomycosis manifests as focal brain lesions, with encapsulated masses present. Mycetoma manifests as deeper tissue lesions. Eumycotic mycetoma, caused by filamentous *Pseudallescheria boydii* and *Madurella grisea*, are organisms that typically drain into sinus tracts with associated swelling of dermal tissue. Other subcutaneous mycoses include rhinosporidiosis (*Rhinosporidium seeberi*), which is a chronic granulomatous disease of mucocutaneous tissue.

Systemic Mycoses

Systemic mycoses are virulent diseases acquired most often through inhalation although they can be acquired by deep trauma. In many cases, they are referred to as fungal pneumonias. Fungi are usually dimorphic, with saprobic forms (deriving energy from organic material in soil) being filamentous and pathogenic forms more characteristic of small, unicellular yeasts. Inhaled spores induce primary responses in lung tissue; symptoms are typically of short duration (Fig. 15-5). Secondary infections are more invasive, with potential spread to other organ systems. The main agents include the pathogens *Histoplasma*, *Coccidioides*, and *Blastomyces*; additional pathogenic organisms will be briefly discussed.

Histoplasma

Inhalation of *Histoplasma capsulatum* hyphae fragments causes histoplasmosis. Saprobic hyphae contain microconidia, and tuberculate macroconidia are readily found in soils with high nitrogen content, such as when contaminated with bird droppings or bat guano. Upon inhalation, small budding yeast forms are phagocytosed, leading to infection of macrophages and histiocytes. Clinically, patients may experience loss of weight and night sweats. A transient spread of disease by infected cells may occur, giving rise to flu-like symptoms. Chronic infection and dissemination of organisms occurs within individuals who have immune defects, leading to prominent hepatosplenomegaly and lesion formation in sites distant from lung tissue.

Blastomyces

Blastomyces dermatitidis is the causative agent of blastomycosis. As a mold, it has characteristic hyphae and microconidia. Upon entry to host lung tissue, it appears as a yeast with a broad-based bud. Primary lung infection is limited in most individuals, controlled via macrophage phagocytosis and subsequent elimination. However, progressive pulmonary disease may occur, with further dissemination to skin or bone, characterized by granulomatous response.

Coccidioides

Coccidioidomycosis, caused by *Coccidioides immitis* and *Coccidioides posadasii*, usually presents as an influenza-like illness with fever, cough, headaches, rash, and myalgias. Some patients do not recover and develop chronic pulmonary infection or widespread disseminated infection (affecting meninges, soft tissues, joints, and bone). Both *C. immitis* and related *C. posadasii* are thermally dimorphic fungi found in soil. Large, round, thick-walled spherules containing endospores are the typical structures formed in infected tissues.

Paracoccidioides

Paracoccidioides brasiliensis is the causative agent of a true systemic (endemic) mycosis called paracoccidioidomycosis. The spectrum of the disease is wide, varying from an asymp-

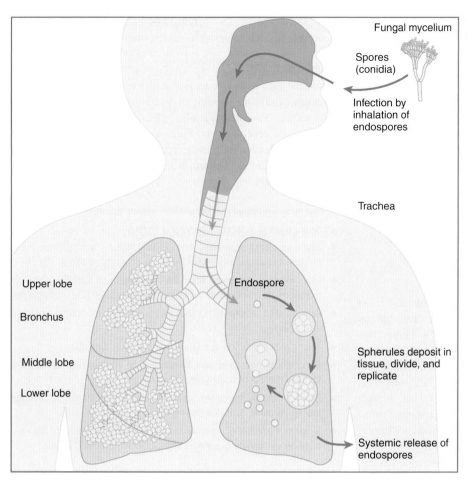

Figure 15-5. General life cycle of systemic mycoses.

tomatic infection verified by the skin test to a subclinical, symptomatic or chronic infection. It is a thermally dimorphic fungus, growing as a mold in soil and as yeast in the host. In addition to the primary pulmonary form of the disease, acute pulmonary, chronic pulmonary, and disseminated forms may also be observed. In cases of disseminated paracoccidioido-mycosis, reticuloendothelial system, skin, and mucous membranes are frequently involved.

Candida

Candida is a yeast and the most common cause of opportunistic mycoses worldwide. It is a frequent colonizer of human skin and mucous membranes and one of the normal flora of skin, mouth, vagina, and stool. Although *Candida albicans* is the most abundant and pathologically significant species among more than 150 identified, *Candida tropicalis, Candida glabrata, Candida parapsilosis, Candida krusei,* and *Candida lusitaniae* also cause *Candida* infections (candidiasis). Disseminated infections arise by hematogenous spread from a primary infected locus. *C. albicans* adheres to host tissues, producing secretory aspartyl proteases and phospholipase enzymes, which contribute to its pathogenicity. Infection may be acquired from exogenous sources (such as catheters or prosthetic devices) or by direct transfer, as seen in oral candidiasis in neonates of mothers with vaginal candidiasis.

Cryptococcus

Cryptococcus is an encapsulated yeast, with more than 35 identified subspecies. *Cryptococcus neoformans* is the causative agent of cryptococcosis, the most common clinical form of which leads to meningoencephalitis. The course of the infection is usually subacute or chronic. Cryptococcosis may also involve the skin, lungs, prostate gland, urinary tract, eyes, myocardium, bones, and joints. Four serotypes have been identified, of which three have been renamed as *Cryptococcus gattii.* The polysaccharide capsule and phenol oxidase enzyme are considered major virulence factors. Infection begins with yeast form inhalation. It is thought that melanizing enzymes from the agent protect the fungal cell from oxidative stress after being engulfed by phagocytic cells.

Aspergillus

Aspergillus fumigatus and other *Aspergillus* spp cause aspergillosis. Aspergillosis produces a variety of symptoms; bronchopulmonary aspergillosis caused by *Aspergillus fumigatus* causes a serve allergic reaction. Aspergilloma is the name given a mycelial ball formed in the lung cavity, causing a person to spit blood; invasive aspergillosis found in immunocompromised persons results in the fungus growing outward from the lungs, invading blood vessels and spreading to other organs. Allergic reactions to fungal antigens are also

Figure 15-6. Aflatoxin B_1. The aflatoxin B_1 (AFB$_1$) is produced by the fungus *Aspergillus flavus*, typically found growing on peanuts. AFB$_1$ is an aromatic amine derivative that is an extremely potent dietary carcinogen having mutagenic effects on hepatocytes.

common. Aflatoxins, such as those produced by *Aspergillus flavus* can lead to severe liver damage (Fig. 15-6).

Mucor

The *Mucor* fungi cause the group of infections referred to as zygomycosis (mucormycosis). *Mucor* is a filamentous fungus found in soil, plants, and decaying fruits. The genus has several species, the more common ones being *Mucor amphibiorum, Mucor circinelloides, Mucor hiemalis, Mucor indicus, Mucor racemosus,* and *Mucor ramosissimus.* Zygomycosis includes mucocutaneous and rhinocerebral infections, as well as septic arthritis, dialysis-associated peritonitis, renal infections, gastritis, and pulmonary infections. Clinical complications arise owing to vascular invasion that causes necrosis of the infected tissue and to perineural invasion.

Morphologically, the organisms are seen as hyphae, sporangiophores, sporangia, and spores.

Pneumocystis

Pneumocystis carinii occurs frequently as an opportunistic infection and also is seen in premature babies and elderly individuals. Symptomatically, infection of lung tissue leads to filling of alveoli with fluids, thus preventing oxygen/gas exchange. Recent sequence analysis of rRNA classifies *P. carinii* as a fungus, moving it out of its historical placement as a protozoan.

KEY POINTS ABOUT MYCOLOGY

- The mycotic species are filamentous, spore-producing eukaryotes including molds, yeasts, and higher fungi.
- The mycotic species may be pathogenic, causing allergic reactions or manifestations of diseases induced by mycotoxins.
- Agents are classified into four major groups according to tissue colonized.
- Superficial mycoses are limited to the skin and hair.
- Cutaneous mycoses are infections of keratinized tissue and include the dermatophytes.
- Subcutaneous mycoses involve infections of subcutaneous fascia, muscle, and deeper epidermal layers.
- Systemic mycoses, usually resulting from inhalation of spores, may be extremely severe in immunocompromised hosts.

Parasitology 16

also be classified according to the role they play in the parasite life cycle. A definitive host is one for which sexual maturity is reached during association, whereas intermediate hosts serve only as temporary reservoirs for physical change (metamorphosis) to another stage. Finally, many pathogens exist within arthropod (or other invertebrate) vectors, serving as an essential component for completion of the parasite life cycle. Parasites of medical importance are listed in Table 16-1.

Almost all interaction with parasites causes histopathology, usually dependent upon numbers of organisms present. In heavy infection, necrosis may occur with death of tissue from persistent immune reactivity to large antigenic loads and assault on parasites. In lesser infections, cellular and tissue swelling may occur, with the increase in cell size due to presence of protein-filled granules. Fatty degeneration may be apparent, with subsequent deposition of large amounts of fat within cells and surrounding tissue. In most cases, infection leads to cellular change, be it hyperplasia or hypertrophy as a result of parasitic stimulation, or metaplasia and neoplasia as cells surrounding parasites are transformed into phenotypes not normally present at sites of infection.

●●● PARASITE PATHOGENESIS

The saying "dead host, dead pathogen" is exemplified in parasitology. By definition, parasites are organisms that shelter within (or on) other organisms and derive benefit from their host. Evolutionary pressures have contributed to establishment of very complex interactions, allowing relatively long periods of host survival with limited pathology so that parasitic life cycles may continue. However, relationships may not always be commensal (mutual parasitism) and may cause diseases such as amebic dysentery, malaria, schistosomiasis, and elephantiasis.

Parasites interact with hosts in many ways. Some organisms are considered symbionts and spend all their life primarily associated with a single host (symbiosis). An obligate parasite is one that can live only in association with its host, whereas a facultative pathogen also can survive in free form. Endoparasites are those parasites capable of living inside the host's body; those that exist on the host body surface are termed ectoparasites. Mutualism is defined as a specialized interaction in which survival depends on physiologic reactions provided by both host and parasite. Hosts may

KEY POINTS ABOUT PARASITES
- Parasites are organisms that shelter within (or on) other organisms, deriving benefit from the host.
- Parasitic organisms may be facultative or require obligate interactions with the host.
- A definitive host is one in which sexual maturity is reached during association.
- Intermediate hosts (or vectors) serve only as temporary reservoirs allowing physical metamorphosis to reach another stage.

●●● PROTOZOA

The protozoa are eukaryotic organisms that are either single-celled or colonial. All have mechanisms of locomotion, whether via flagella (Fig. 16-1), allowing transport in fluid (blood or lymph), or through pseudopodia, as seen in amoebae. Pseudopodia (filopodia, axopodia, rhizopodia, and lobopodia) allow mobility along substrates, but unlike the flagella, do not assist in swimming within fluids.

TABLE 16-1. Medically Important Parasites

Intestinal Protozoa
  Balantidium coli
  Blastocystis hominis
  Chilomastix mesnili
  Cryptosporidium spp
  Cyclospora spp
  Dientamoeba fragilis
  Eimeria tenella
  Entamoeba coli
  Entamoeba histolytica
  Endolimax nana
  Giardia lamblia
  Iodamoeba bütschlii
  Trichomonas hominis
Nematodes
  Ancylostoma duodenale
  Ascaris lumbricoides
  Enterobius vermicularis
  Necator americanus
  Strongyloides stercoralis
  Toxocara canis
  Trichinella spiralis
  Trichuris trichiura
Extraintestinal Protozoa
  Acanthamoeba spp
  Babesia microti
  Entamoeba gingivalis
  Eimeria stiedai
  Giardia duodenalis
  Histomonas meleagridis
  Leishmania spp

  Naegleria fowleri
  Plasmodium spp
  Pneumocystis carinii
  Toxoplasma gondii
  Trichomonas vaginalis
  Trypanosoma spp
Cestodes and Trematodes
  Clonorchis sinensis
  Diphyllobothrium latum
  Echinococcus granulosus
  Echinostoma revolutum
  Fasciola hepatica
  Fasciolopsis buski
  Hymenolepis spp
  Moniezia expansa
  Paragonimus westermani
  Schistosoma spp
  Taenia spp
Filariae
  Brugia malayi
  Dirofilaria immitis
  Loa loa
  Onchocerca volvulus
  Wuchereria bancrofti
Lice and Mites
  Dermatophagoides spp
  Eutrombicula alfreddugesi
  Pediculus humanus
  Pthirus pubis
  Sarcoptes scabiei

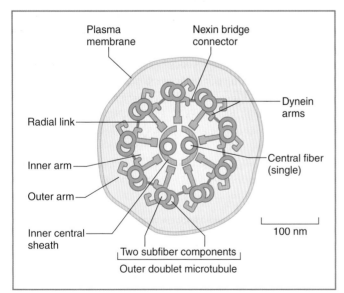

Figure 16-1. Flagellar organization. A flagellum (pl. *flagella*) is an extension of ectoplasm that moves in a whip-like manner to provide locomotion for unicellular protozoa. The basic structure is that of longitudinal cilium composed of microtubules arranged in nine doublets with two complete doublets in the center.

The protozoa have nuclei as well as defined mitochondria and Golgi complex components. Indeed, certain protozoa possess acid hydrolase–filled lysosomes that assist degradation of phagocytosed food particles. Common means of reproduction include asexual binary fission, as seen in amoebae, flagellates, and ciliates. Alternatively, schizogony (multiple fission) can occur, as seen with *Plasmodium* (malaria) in which multinucleated cells appear (schizonts) followed by breaking off of single-cell merozoites. In many cases (such as with merozoites) asexual replication may continue, or organisms may undergo further transformation to differentiated gametocytes for sexual reproduction.

ANATOMY

Reproduction of Higher Eukaryotes

Reproduction of complex eukaryotes involves the union of two unlike sex cells (gametes), the sperm and the ovum, followed by the joining of their nuclei to form a zygote. This begins a rapid series of cell divisions (mitosis) in which segmentation occurs, giving rise to a hollow ball one cell thick, called a blastula.

Intestinal Protozoa

The intestinal protozoa are aptly named, causing clinical complications of dysentery due to residence in the lower gastrointestinal tract of the host. The common infective form is a cyst, usually transmitted by ingestion of contaminated food or water. In general, cysts modify their structure inside the host (excystation) to become trophozoites, which are the reproductive and feeding forms of the organism.

KEY POINTS ABOUT PROTOZOA

- Intestinal protozoa are causative agents of gastrointestinal disorders.
- Extraintestinal protozoa disseminate within the host to alternate sites, leading to varied pathology and tissue damage.

Amebae

Entamoeba histolytica is the major pathogenic intestinal protozoan and the cause of amebic dysentery in humans. It is a nonpathogenic commensal that is transmitted via a cyst stage through contact with infected feces or foods. Many other related amebae belonging to this group are nonpatho-

HISTOLOGY

Histologic Organization of the Colon

The main function of the colon is fluid absorption and concentration of solid waste. The inner tunica mucosa contains specialized epithelial cells and glands (goblet cells) and a thin muscularis mucosae underlying the lamina propria. A submucosal layer with lymphatic nodules is surrounded by a muscularis externa, comprising outer longitudinal and inner circular muscle layers. The entire organ is contained by an overlying serosa.

genic; e.g., *Entamoeba coli* is a commensal that is commonly mistaken for *E. histolytica*. A general life cycle is depicted in Figure 16-2.

Ciliates

Balantidium coli is a pathogenic ciliate that is the largest of the parasitic protozoans and responsible for balantidial dysentery. Infection is acquired through ingestion of cysts from fecally contaminated water. *Balantidium* is partially invasive, causing intestinal lesions along submucosal tissue. Cyst forms excystate into trophozoites that multiply by binary fission.

Flagellates

Intestinal flagellates include pathogenic *Giardia lamblia* and *Dientamoeba fragilis*, as well as multiple nonpathogenic species. *Giardia*, one of the causative agents of traveler's diarrhea, and *Dientamoeba* are transmitted via infected food or placement of contaminated fingers in the oral cavity. The life cycle of *Giardia* is similar to that of amebae (described above) with infective multinucleated cysts in feces ingested, and excystation to a trophozoite form (Fig. 16-3). *Dientamoeba* has a double-nucleated trophozoite stage but no known cyst form.

Coccidia

Cryptosporidium parvum and *Cyclospora* spp are coccidian parasites that cause self-limiting diarrhea. The incidence of reported infections has increased in recent years, especially in immunocompromised individuals. The general life cycle begins with the definitive host ingesting oocysts containing eight sporozoites. Once inside the intestine, developing merozoites within the schizont form are released to enter intestinal epithelium and begin the sexual cycle phase. Sexual union (gametogony) produces an oocyst, with oocytes subsequently released to the environment. Because of intermittent findings in stool samples, positive diagnosis requires

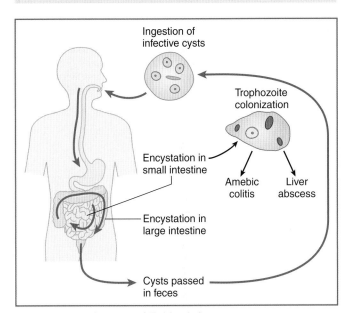

Figure 16-2. Life cycle of *E. histolytica*.

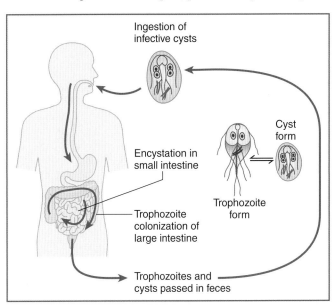

Figure 16-3. Life cycle of *Giardia*.

examination of three fecal specimens collected on alternate days. The oocysts of *Cyclospora* (8–10 µM) are roughly twice the size of *Cryptosporidium* oocytes (4 µM). In immunocompromised patients, *Cryptosporidium* may also inhabit respiratory and biliary tract tissue.

The cat is thought to be the definitive host for *Toxoplasma gondii*, in which it resides as an intestinal parasite. In humans, *T. gondii* is an extraintestinal coccidian parasite that infects and undergoes schizogony in nucleated cells. *Toxoplasma* divides mitotically in humans as tachyzoites, giving rise to groups of organisms (pseudocysts or bradyzoites) that may reside in tissue sites (brain, heart, or skeletal muscles). Bradyzoite clusters may eventually become encysted, coinciding with developing immune responses. Toxoplasmosis is a common opportunistic infection associated with AIDS; weakened immune systems allow emergence from cysts to cause further tissue damage. Pregnant women who are carrying their first child are warned to limit exposure to cats to reduce infection potential and harm to the fetus.

Extraintestinal Protozoa

Extraintestinal protozoa include many organisms that are spread by vector agents. Many parasitic diseases are found throughout the tropical regions of the world; however, the distribution of various organisms is changing with increasing human travel. Whereas the intestinal protozoa were major contributions of intestine-related disorders, the pathologies associated with extraintestinal protozoa are more diverse owing to the nature of organism dissemination and complex interactions at multiple tissue sites.

Plasmodium

There are more than 150 identified species of *Plasmodium*, the causative agent of malaria. Four species are known to infect human hosts: *Plasmodium falciparum*, *Plasmodium vivax*, *Plasmodium ovale*, and *Plasmodium malariae*. The life cycle is complex, and includes morphologic changes in both the human and the mosquito (*Anopheles*) host (Fig. 16-4). Clinical presentation is dependent upon the infecting species; however, all produce symptoms including fever and chills, headache and myalgias, and anemia. Infections caused by *P. falciparum* can be severe and fatal, with occurrence of central nervous system (CNS) inflammation (cerebral malaria) and accompanying acute renal failure. Travelers to endemic areas should limit exposure and use insect repellants and prophylaxis. Mefloquine, doxycycline, and chloroquine are effective antimalarial agents.

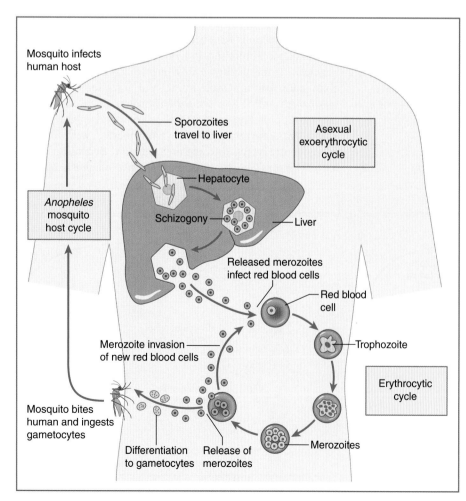

Figure 16-4. Life cycle of *Plasmodium* (malaria). The *Plasmodium* life cycle involves human and mosquito (*Anopheles*) hosts. Human hosts are infected by mosquitoes during a blood meal, following which sporozoites infect hepatocytes. Maturing schizonts split open hepatocytes, causing release of merozoites, which go on to infect RBCs. RBCs from ring-stage trophozoites mature into schizonts. Alternatively, trophozoites can mature into gametocytes, which may be ingested by mosquitoes during feeding. Multiplication in the mosquito host leads to a series of morphologic changes resulting in sporozoite formation for infection of humans, thus completing the life cycle.

Babesia

Babesiosis is a malaria-like illness caused by a protozoan parasite *Babesia microti* or other species members. Symptoms of infection include gradual onset of malaise and fatigue, followed by headaches, muscle pain, and high fever. The parasite is transmitted primarily by *Ixodes* ticks (deer ticks) and invades red blood cells (RBCs). Care must be taken in the examination of blood smears to not confuse *Babesia* spp with *Plasmodium*, since both exhibit ring forms in RBCs.

Trypanosoma

Trypanosoma cruzi, or Chagas disease, is transmitted to humans by blood-sucking triatomine bugs (kissing bugs), releasing trypomastigotes in its feces near the blood-meal wound. Trypomastigotes transform into amastigotes that multiply by binary fission in infected tissue. Clinical manifestations begin with a local lesion at the site of inoculation, with accompanying inflammation and edema. Self-resolving acute-stage symptoms include low fever, lymphadenopathy, and slight hepatosplenomegaly. Late (chronic) infection occurs many years after initial infection and can lead to progressive encephalitis and dementia and myocarditis. Organs of the digestive tract may also be affected. Related protozoan hemoflagellates, *Trypanosoma brucei gambiense* and *Trypanosoma brucei rhodesiense*, are causative agents of sleeping sickness common to West and East Africa. These agents are spread by the tsetse fly (*Glossina*), with CNS involvement and dementia seen in late-stage disease.

Leishmania

Leishmaniasis is caused by the obligate intracellular protozoan *Leishmania*, of which more than 20 different species are known to induce human disease. The organism is transmitted by sandflies. *Leishmania donovani*, *Leishmania mexicana*, *Leishmania tropica*, and *Leishmania major* are major causes of disease. Each species is somewhat distinct and can be identified serologically. Upon a blood meal, promastigotes are transferred to the human host; promastigotes develop inside macrophages. There are two main forms of disease: cutaneous leishmaniasis and visceral leishmaniasis (also called kala-azar). Cutaneous leishmaniasis is characterized by skin lesions, whereas kala-azar presents as a more severe disease with hepatosplenomegaly and loss of white blood cells.

Trichomonas

Trichomonas vaginalis is a flagellated protozoan that replicates in the genitourinary tract of males and females. It is not carried by vector arthropods but rather is spread by sexual intercourse and contact. It does not form cysts but has a characteristic trophozoite form with a large nucleus, four anterior flagella, and an undulating membrane. Treatment with a single dose of metronidazole is sufficient to clear infection.

Acanthamoeba and Naegleria

Acanthamoeba spp and *Naegleria fowleri* are free living, freshwater amebae that cause a potentially lethal CNS disease referred to as primary amebic meningoencephalitis. The *Acanthamoeba* spp are similar to *Entamoeba*; however, infection leads to a more chronic form of disease, identified by pathologic manifestations of chronic granulomatous encephalitis. *N. fowleri* trophozoites infect humans by entering the olfactory neuroepithelium, eventually reaching the brain to cause disease with CNS involvement. *Balamuthia mandrillaris* is a related organism that may cause disease in immunocompromised individuals.

●●● NEMATODES

The nematodes are commonly referred to as roundworms. They range in size from millimeter length to over a meter. The male is typically smaller than the female. One end of the parasite has an attachment appendage, such as oral hooks or plates within the oral cavity (buccal capsule). The body is covered by a surface cuticle (Fig. 16-5).

Pinworms and Whipworms

Enterobiasis (pinworms, *Enterobius vermicularis*) and trichuriasis (whipworms, *Trichuris trichiura*) can be acquired through environmental contact with soil or food contaminated with eggs. The infective eggs are ingested, and the larvae hatch within the small intestine. The adult worms live in the cecum and ascending colon. For pinworm, the adult female worm is slightly larger (8–12 cm) than the male (3–5 cm); the adult whipworms are roughly 4 cm in length. Clinically, infection is manifested as abdominal pain and diarrhea, resulting from reactivity to egg deposition; females can shed between 3000 and 20,000 eggs per day.

Ascaris

Ascariasis, caused by *Ascaris lumbricoides*, is the largest roundworm able to parasitize the human intestine (up to 30–35 cm in length). The human infection cycle begins with ingestion of infective eggs, following which hatched larvae first invade the mucosa of the intestine and are then carried through lymphatics to the portal vein and finally to the lungs. The larvae mature in the lungs, penetrate the alveolar walls, and ascend the bronchial tree to the throat, where they are swallowed. Adult worms mature in the small intestine, where

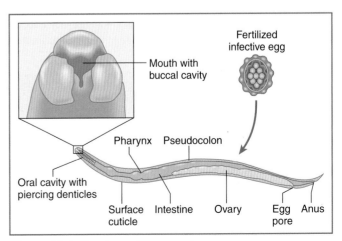

Figure 16-5. Structure of the roundworm.

the female reportedly can lay up to 200,000 eggs per day. The eggs are passed from the host with the feces. *Ascaris* infection is the most common nematode infection; treatment with albendazole or mebendazole is successful.

Hookworm

The two roundworm nematode species, *Ancylostoma duodenale* and *Necator americanus*, are the causative agents of hookworm. Filariform larvae physically penetrate the skin and are carried through the veins to the heart and lungs, eventually ascending the bronchial tree to the pharynx, where they are swallowed. Maturation to the adult form is accomplished in the small intestine, where adult worms mate and produce eggs. An early clinical feature of infection is that of cutaneous larva migrans, a form of acquired dermatosis that occurs during skin penetration and migration of organisms to other tissue sites. Blood loss through destruction of intestinal tissue is a common clinical feature of chronic infection.

Strongyloides

Strongyloidiasis is caused by the intestinal nematodes *Strongyloides stercoralis* and *Strongyloides fuelleborni*. Infective filariform larvae penetrate soil-exposed skin. Larvae travel to lung tissue, enter airways, and are swallowed. Adult worms mature in the intestines, and females begin to lay eggs. Eggs hatch in the intestinal tract to produce rhabditiform larvae. Larvae may be released to the soil where free-living adults can mate and lay eggs. Alternatively, larvae may be available for autoinfection and continuation of the infective cycle. Although *Strongyloides* is an intestinal nematode, the larvae can spread to the respiratory tract, resulting in hemoptysis and pulmonary infiltrates. The organism is eosinophilic on Papanicolaou (Pap) stains and ranges from 400 to 500 µm in length in cytologic preparations. Its internal structure, a closed gullet, and V-shaped notched tail are characteristic for diagnostic purposes. Treatment is usually with albendazole or thiabendazole.

Trichinella

Trichinellosis (trichinosis) is caused by the nematode *Trichinella spiralis*, acquired by eating cyst-contaminated meat (typically uncooked pork). Released larvae enter the intestinal mucosa and develop into adult male and female worms. The cycle continues as larvae released from adult worms enter the lymphatics and mesenteric veins, travel to the heart and lungs, and then enter the arterial system, which distributes them throughout the body. The final stage is entry to striated muscle, where they penetrate fibers and encyst. Viable cysts can survive for decades within the host. Clinical symptoms include initial gastrointestinal disorders (nausea, diarrhea, abdominal pain) and chronic complications due to larval migration and encystations in muscle tissues. Diagnosis may be made by muscle biopsy or by screening for antibodies to pathogenic antigens.

Filariae

Filarial pathogenesis (filariasis) is due to the presence of filaria-stage organisms in the circulation and most often is characterized by inflammation of the lymphatic vessels. Three specific organisms are major causes of disease: *Wuchereria bancrofti* and *Brugia malayi* cause lymphatic filariasis, and *Onchocerca volvulus* causes river blindness (onchocerciasis). Other species also cause pathogenesis, including *Loa loa*. The clinical manifestations include extreme lymphedema and elephantiasis, in large part due to immune reactions within draining lymphatics that occlude vessels.

The life cycle of filariae begins with the arthropod vector (mosquito, midge, or blackfly) spreading infection during a blood meal. The larvae migrate to the appropriate site of the host's body, where they develop into adults. Females produce microfilarial offspring that circulate in the blood, skin, or eye (in the case of *O. volvulus*) and can migrate to subcutaneous tissue. It is critical to understand life cycle stages and periodicity of the microfilariae when considering diagnosis. Blood stages can be identified by smear staining, but skin snips also are a useful tool for detection of microfilariae.

●●● CESTODES AND TREMATODES
Taenia and *Echinococcus*

The cestodes include *Taenia saginata* (the beef tapeworm) and *Taenia solium* (the pork tapeworm) and *Echinococcus granulosus* (the hydatid worm). Both *Taenia* spp have similar life cycles and eggs that are morphologically indistinguishable. Pigs serve as the intermediate host for *T. solium*; humans are infected when they ingest an immature tapeworm (a cysticercus) in undercooked pork, leading to harboring of adult sexually active worms within the intestinal tract. However, if humans ingest *T. solium* eggs, hatching cysticerci lead to cysticercosis. In this case, larvae produced in the small intestine migrate to other tissues. Resulting cyst forms may lead to tissue-related disease, such as neurocysticercosis when brain tissue is affected.

E. granulosus is the cestode tapeworm agent responsible for causing cystic echinococcosis, a cystic disease that can have a strong hepatic obstructive component in human infection. The human is an intermediate host, with members of the canine

---

PATHOLOGY

Cutaneous Larva Migrans

Cutaneous larva migrans is a parasitic skin disease caused by filarial hookworm larvae that penetrate human skin and then migrate subcutaneously, leaving extremely itchy red lines that may be accompanied by blisters (also called "creeping eruption" or "ground itch"). The reaction is characterized by erythematous, serpiginous (having wavy white-dotted lesions with indented margins), and pruritic dermatitis.

species being the definitive host. Also known as "hydatid worm," related members of the genus are known to cause alveolar echinococcosis and polycystic echinococcosis. Eggs ingested by an intermediate host hatch into larvae that travel through the blood and form hydatid cysts in the host's tissues (liver, lung, or brain). In the definitive host, the larvae transform into full tapeworms, which pass infective eggs in the feces.

Schistosomes

Three main species of *Schistosoma* trematodes are the causative agents for schistosomiasis. They are *Schistosoma haematobium*, *Schistosoma japonicum,* and *Schistosoma mansoni.* The schistosomal life cycle is depicted in Figure 16-6. Eggs released environmentally with feces hatch, and resulting miracidia infect a freshwater snail vector. Free-swimming cercariae released from the snail infect humans wading through infected waters, using an elastase to bore into the skin of the host. Cercariae will transform to schistosome form, travel to lung tissue, and eventually come to reside in the portal blood, where they develop into adult male and female worms. Specifically, *S. mansoni* and *S. japonicum* are frequently found in the superior mesenteric veins draining the large and small intestine, respectively, whereas *S. haematobium* often invades the bladder venous plexus. In all cases, organisms may reside in multiple tissue sites.

Damaging pathology ensues from immune responses to the eggs, with a resultant granulomatous response. A characteristic occurrence during infection is eosinophilia, thought to be induced by specific interleukins released by a skewed T-cell response. Over time heavy fibrosis, calcification, and tissue scarring occur, often resembling cross-sectioning of a pipe stem, leading to hepatic enlargement and severe hypertension. Clinical symptoms of hematuria and squamous cell carcinoma are common. Praziquantel and oxamniquine historically have been effective for treatment of disease-causing pathogens.

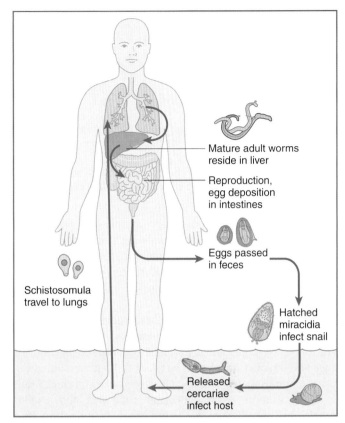

Figure 16-6. Life cycle of *Schistosoma*.

HISTOLOGY

Liver

The liver is a filter for toxic metabolites. The parenchyma comprises liver plates (hepatocytes) with endothelial cells establishing sinusoids for blood flow. The characteristic portal triad contains at least one profile each of a hepatic artery, a portal vein, and an interlobular bile duct.

KEY POINTS ABOUT NEMATODES, CESTODES, AND TREMATODES

- The nematodes (roundworms) are generally large parasites that generate adult worms producing larvae or eggs that are damaging to the host.
- Cestodes and trematodes include the tapeworms and schistosomes, respectively.
- In all cases, adult worms give rise to eggs and/or cysts that cause physical damage, in part due to immunologic responsiveness to foreign antigens.

●●● LICE AND MITES

Humans are hosts to the head louse (*Pediculus humanus capitis*), the body louse (*Pediculus humanus humanus*), and the crab louse (*Pthirus pubis*). Lice attach to hair shafts and lay eggs (nits). Lice derive nutrients through tissue by blood-feeding and cause itching and irritation (Fig. 16-7). They are readily treatable with over-the-counter chemical applications.

Mites are related to ticks and spiders. There are many species, with commonalities in biting and bloodsucking behavior causing irritation and discomfort; many species are also known to elicit allergic reactions. Mites are spread by direct contact. Common mites that affect human hosts include *Sarcoptes scabiei* (scabies), *Eutrombicula alfreddugesi* (chiggers), and *Dermatophagoides pteronyssinus* and *Dermatophagoides farinae* (house dust mites). Treatment can be as simple as administration of oral antihistamines and application of hydrocortisone cream to relieve associated symptoms.

●●● LABORATORY DIAGNOSIS OF PARASITIC INFECTIONS

Identification of parasites is critical for proper treatment and limitation of pathology within the host. Knowledge of the characteristics of clinically significant human parasites

A   B

Figure 16-7. A, The common head and body louse (*Pediculus humanus*). **B,** The crab louse (*Pthirus pubis*).

includes recognition of organism morphology at various stages of life cycles and understanding the relationship of morphology to disease state. In addition, the medical practitioner must understand potential routes of infection and appreciate the value of appropriate clinical specimen collection to diagnosis of disease.

Many diagnoses begin with macroscopic examination of fecal material, with regard to consistency of stool specimen and presence of intestinal protozoa or visual inspection for eggs and larvae. Care should be taken to limit contamination from environmental sources and from patient urine. Adult worms are more easily detectable than ova and smaller organisms, which require microscopic examination and separation of stool into components for identification by staining techniques. The Wheatley trichrome technique is a rapid way to stain for intestinal protozoa, allowing identification of cysts. *Cryptosporidium* is more easily identified with a modified Kinyoun acid-fast stain. Pinworms lay eggs in the perianal region and may be recovered using a simple cellophane tape method. For blood-borne parasites, serology is the simplest means of detection. Although culture of organisms is usually possible, detection of host antibodies against different-stage proteins reveals information on tissue migration and developmental stage and may also indicate relative numbers and activity of infection. Standard enzyme-linked immunosorbent assays (ELISAs) are a quick way to determine current or past exposure and are available for most common pathogens. Finally, blood smears are a rapid way to determine presence of schizogony for organisms such as *Plasmodium, Babesia, Leishmania,* and *Trypanosoma.* Fixed peripheral blood is treated with Giemsa stain to allow visualization of intracellular parasites or of microfilariae.

●●● IMMUNE RESPONSE TO PARASITIC INFECTIONS

Host immune responses to parasitic infections are dictated by organism size, location within the host, and parasite complexity. For example, the immune response to intestinal protozoa is primarily humoral and inflammatory. Protozoa such as *Cryptosporidium* and the *Entamoeba* spp stimulate an immune response from the gut-associated lymphoid tissue. Initial reactivity begins with a nidus of tissue damage and ensuing activation of enterocytes, characterized by release of cytokines and chemokines. In turn, dendritic cells and macrophages (antigen-presenting cells) initiate recognition by lymphocytes. In most cases, lymphocytes induce production of proinflammatory responses while triggering B cells to produce both IgA and IgG antibody subclasses.

Extraintestinal protozoa represent further requirements for complexity in immune responses. The malaria parasite changes morphology during its life cycle in humans, which requires different immune interventions. While blood-stage protection can be mediated by antibodies, a T-cell and productive interferon response against blood-stage antigens may be required for complete protection against disease. *Toxoplasma* is an organism that easily crosses encephalic and placental barriers. The limited acute phase of this infection is associated with strong interferon responses elicited from T lymphocytes, effectively limiting tissue dissemination. However, this specific lymphocyte response triggers an organism life-cycle change resulting in manifestation as an intracellular bradyzoite that may persist in brain and muscle tissue. Trypanosomes bring about an even more complex response. Primary resolution of trypanosomal infection is through antibody recognition of surface antigens; variations in surface glycoproteins through molecular rearrangement of DNA sequences allow replicating organisms to escape specific host antibody recognition.

Nematodes, cestodes, and trematodes undergo physical changes as they adapt to life in the host, and they are therefore subject to differing immune mechanisms dependent upon form (larval, adult, or egg stage). Tissue reaction to *Ascaris* and *Trichinella* consists of an intense infiltrate of polymorphonuclear leukocytes, with a predominance of eosinophils. Likewise, schistosomes are readily attacked by eosinophils and mast cells, through complex stimulation patterns released by both T cells and antibody-dependent cell cytotoxicity (ADCC). Proteins reacting with IgE antibody bound to intestinal mast cells stimulate release of inflammatory mediators, such as histamine, proteases, leukotrienes, prostaglandins, and serotonin. However, schistosomal eggs trigger responses from macrophages and T cells, leading to development of a granulomatous physical encapsulation of slowly released, nondigestible antigenic materials.

KEY POINTS ABOUT PARASITOLOGY

- It is extremely important to understand the life cycle and have strong knowledge of developmental stages of parasites for positive diagnostic identification to occur.
- Immunologic mechanisms to combat parasite pathogens are varied, dependent upon size and number of organisms and relative location of directed responses.

Case Studies

CASE STUDY 1

A 14-year-old Hispanic male was admitted to the emergency room with complaints of centered abdominal pain that progressed to the right lower quadrant. Additional symptoms included vomiting and slight diarrhea. Physical examination revealed tenderness with guarding (muscle tensing) upon touch. Blood tests showed slightly elevated white blood cell (WBC) count of 16,300/mm^3 (normal, <12,000/μL). A diagnosis of appendicitis (inflammation of the appendix) was made, and appendectomy was immediately performed.

1. **What is the function of the appendix?**

2. **What is the common cause of appendicitis?**

3. **What are complications if appendicitis is left untreated?**

CASE STUDY 2

An 11-month-old male presents with rapid onset of high fever and elevated WBC count due to an upper respiratory infection of *Haemophilus influenzae*. The child has a history of recurrent bacterial infections with encapsulated organisms. Upon clinical examination, the spleen was not palpable. A diagnosis of congenital asplenia was made.

1. **How does the lack of a spleen affect immune cell function, and what implications does this have for immune responses to infective agents?**

2. **Why does loss of a spleen represent more of a clinical problem in children than in adults?**

3. **What is the appropriate medical care and response for congenital asplenia?**

CASE STUDY 3

A 12-year old female gymnast developed pain in her upper right thigh, which increased progressively during stretching prior to floor exercise competition. During competition, she landed incorrectly and broke her leg. Radiographs reveal a fractured femur; however, spongy appearing lesions are also seen throughout her leg long bones. Laboratory analysis shows a mild anemia and neutropenia with decreased WBC count of 3200/mL (normal, 5000/mL) and highly elevated IgG levels at 4250 mg/dL (normal, 700–1000 mg/dL). The diagnosis is multiple myeloma, and she is started on a chemotherapeutic regimen.

1. **What is the immunologic basis for multiple myeloma?**

2. **What is the pathologic basis for the spongy appearance of bone tissue?**

3. **In the face of high antibody levels, why are patients considered more susceptible to bacterial infections?**

CASE STUDY 4

An 8-month-old male presents to the pediatrician with recurrent ear and sinus infections. Physical examination reveals distinctive downward-slanting eyes; low-set, rotated ears; and a small, round mouth. Radiographs and computed tomography scans demonstrate absence of a thymic shadow. Laboratory analysis of WBCs reveals chromosomal defects, and the child is given the diagnosis of DiGeorge syndrome.

1. **What is the pathologic basis of DiGeorge syndrome?**

2. **What is the effect of thymus absence on maturation of T cells?**

3. **What is the prognosis for patients with DiGeorge syndrome?**

CASE STUDY 5

A 53-year old black male with a history of emphysema underwent a single lung organ transplant. He has been on a cyclosporine and corticosteroid–based regimen to limit possibilities of graft rejection. His postoperative course had been unremarkable until the recent development of a cough with production of heavy yellow sputum.

He complains of increasing fatigue but does not have night sweats, fever, or chills. Rhonchi (leathery wheezing) can be heard within the transplanted lung; a radiograph reveals extensive interstitial infiltrates. A bronchoscopic biopsy specimen does not show evidence of rejection, nor is there evidence of granulomas (a chronic inflamed tissue mass). However, viral inclusions are apparent, and the eventual diagnosis is parainfluenza as the cause of the upper respiratory infection and bronchitis.

1. **How do immunosuppressive drugs contribute to the pathology seen in this case?**

2. **What is the molecular basis for graft rejection in patients receiving donor tissue?**

3. **What other viral associations are commonly found in transplant patients?**

CASE STUDY 6

A 14-month-old male is brought to the pediatrician because of a deep and painful perirectal abscess. His WBC count is greater than 45,000 (normal, less than 10,000), and his spleen is enlarged (splenomegaly). His parents and siblings are healthy. Lymphocyte function, antibody formation, nitroblue tetrazolium test (NBT), and complement function are normal. Further examination of WBC populations reveals a deficiency in chemotactic activity, and a diagnosis of leukocyte adhesion deficiency (LAD) is made.

1. **What is the molecular basis for LAD?**

2. **What is the function of the NBT test?**

3. **What is the prognosis for LAD?**

CASE STUDY 7

A 4-month-old female is referred to City Hospital after 3 weeks of prolonged fever episodes and sores in the upper mouth and on the tongue. Immunophenotypic analysis of blood cells identifies a marked eosinophilia and a deficiency in the mature T lymphocyte and B lymphocyte population. In addition, serum antibody levels are low for all immunoglobulin isotypes. Proliferative responses to mitogens (concanavalin A and lipopolysaccharide) are markedly reduced. Based on clinical, immunologic, and genetic findings, Omenn syndrome is diagnosed.

1. **What is the molecular basis for Omenn's syndrome?**

2. **Why do patients with Omenn's syndrome demonstrate eosinophilia?**

3. **What is the prognosis for Omenn's syndrome?**

CASE STUDY 8

A 34-year-old male complained of the sudden onset of weakness in the extremities, coincident with increased work-related stress. The patient demonstrated a slightly elevated WBC count but no increase in banded patterns (polymorphonuclear cells) and no fever. Culture tests did not identify a causative infectious agent. Symptoms resolved with rest and return to normal routine. Now, 5 years later, after an especially stressful month of work, the symptoms returned with noticeable loss of upper arm strength and awkwardness in gait. WBC count is elevated, with right shift indicative of increased lymphocytic responses. The increased neurologic dysfunction warrants an MRI, upon which evidence of plaque formation in the CNS is found. Early-stage multiple sclerosis is diagnosed.

1. **What is the immunologic basis for multiple sclerosis?**

2. **What is meant by the diagnostic indication of plaques?**

3. **What factors contribute to development of MS?**

CASE STUDY 9

A 19-year-old college student complains of shortness of breath, swollen gums, and persistent fever. He also indicates that he bruises easily, at times with no apparent cause, and reports abnormally long times for cuts to heal. Close examination of skin tissue reveals small petechial hemorrhages under the skin. Blood tests lead to the diagnosis of acute myelogenous leukemia (AML). He immediately undergoes extensive and aggressive radiation therapy and chemotherapy. He receives a bone marrow transplant from a sibling and is given a short course of immunosuppressive therapeutics.

1. What is AML?

2. What are possible side effects of bone marrow transplantation?

3. What are the ABO blood group antigens?

4. Why was the patient given a course of immunosuppressive therapeutics?

CASE STUDY 10

A 16-year-old Chinese female awoke with slight fever. She took two aspirins and went to school; however, by mid-morning she had a diffuse macular erythroderma (rash) on her extremities. A noninvasive examination by the school nurse indicated no abnormal use of drugs or alcohol; however, it was readily apparent that she was disoriented and in need of emergency care. En route to the ER, she complained of severe myalgia (muscle pain) and lost consciousness owing to hypotension. Laboratory tests indicated elevated creatine phosphokinase (CPK) and alanine aminotransferase (ALT) levels, and pyuria (pus in the urine). *Staphylococcus aureus* was isolated from blood cultures. Toxic shock syndrome is diagnosed.

1. What is toxic shock syndrome?

2. What is the immunologic basis for toxic shock?

3. What was the basis of her physical symptoms?

CASE STUDY 11

A 76-year-old male is admitted to the emergency room for treatment of cellulitis on the top of his left foot and the appearance of a blistering hematoma (5 × 5 cm) with radiating erythema on his left heel. CBC studies reveal a left shift, with elevated WBC count of 23,800/mm^3 (normal, <12,000/μL). The radiograph of the ankle and foot shows extensive gas in the soft tissues. A biopsy specimen taken from the wound area reveals few neutrophils in spite of the high WBC count. On gram-positive staining, boxcar-shaped rods are identified that do not grow on aerobic cultures.

1. Which organism is responsible for the disease?

2. Which factors contribute to the pathology?

3. What is the course of action for treatment?

CASE STUDY 12

A 49-year-old female caseworker for child protective services complains of persistent cough, night sweats, loss of appetite and weight, and occasional blood-streaked sputum. The patient has a 20-year history of smoking (one pack per day). Cardiopulmonary examination is unremarkable. WBC count is slightly elevated at 16,700/mm^3 (normal, 4500–10,500/mm^3), but blood chemistry levels are within normal range. Chest radiograph reveals lung infiltrate, and a CT scan confirms thick-walled cavitation in the upper right lobe. Acid-fast organisms grow from cultured sputum and bronchoalveolar lavage (BAL) fluid, and are identified as *Mycobacterium tuberculosis*.

1. What is the immunologic basis for the lung cavitation?

2. Which factors in the patient's history contribute to disease-related pathology?

3. What therapeutic intervention is prescribed for this individual?

4. Why do these organisms stain acid fast?

CASE STUDY 13

An otherwise healthy 29-year-old white female presents with a 3-day history of headaches, fever, stiff neck, and photophobia (painful sensitivity to light). She shows general malaise and lethargy. The patient also indicates nausea with two incidents of vomiting, and watery diarrhea persisting for almost a week. She has no history of sexually transmitted diseases and is HIV-negative. A lumbar puncture is performed, revealing lymphocytic pleocytosis (increased cellularity) in the cerebrospinal fluid (CSF). Polymerase chain reaction (PCR) and antibody reactivity tests reveal that she suffers from aseptic meningitis occurring from reactivated herpes simplex virus 2 (HSV-2) infection.

1. What is the likely history of this patient?

2. What effects does HSV-2 have on the brain and CNS?

3. Which events led to reactivation of infection?

CASE STUDY 14

A 28-year old Hispanic male presents to City Hospital with right-lower-quadrant abdominal crampy pain, recent excessive weight loss, fever, fatigue, and nonbloody diarrhea. The patient denies intravenous drug use or homosexual activity, but he admits to recently serving 2 years in the county jail. He has multiple tattoos and a history of stab wounds. Laboratory tests indicate the patient is HIV-positive, and he admits to being noncompliant with HAART therapy. He has a viral load of >300,000 copies/mL and a CD4 count of approximately 120. He is PPD-negative at the time of testing. A CT scan of the abdomen shows thickening of the cecum and ascending colon but no lymphadenopathy.

1. **Which organism(s) might be responsible for the disease?**

2. **What is the course of action for treatment?**

3. **What is HAART therapy?**

CASE STUDY 15

A 40-day-old female neonate born 6 weeks premature underwent corrective surgery to remove an oral cyst. The surgery was successful; however, 4 days later the infant has fever, tachycardia (rapid heart rate), tachypnea (increased respiration rate), and thrombocytopenia (decreased blood platelets). The area around a percutaneously inserted central line appears swollen and red with obvious phlebitis (inflammation of vein). Blood cultures taken from the central line are positive for *Candida albicans*; the child is immediately started on antifungal therapeutics and improvement in her condition is noticed shortly thereafter.

1. **What are predisposing risk factors for candidiasis in the neonate?**

2. **What is the likely source of contamination for this child?**

3. **What are complications if the fungal infection is not treated effectively and immediately?**

CASE STUDY 16

A 35-year-old male living in the Blue Ridge Mountains of Tennessee comes in with right-upper-quadrant pain, slight nausea, and a 2-week history of diarrhea. Visual examination shows calloused hands, the presence of tattoos on his right forearm, and a slight yellowish tint to his sclera. He is a Honduran immigrant who has been in the United States for 6 years. He admits to alcohol consumption of at least two beers per day and indicates he spent 8 months in prison in 2002. He is PPD-negative and HIV-negative. Blood tests show an elevated leukocyte count of 7600/mm^3, with 54% neutrophils (within normal range) and 12% eosinophils (highly elevated).

1. **Which organ systems are affected, and what could be the possible cause of the disorder?**

2. **What complications are associated with this type of infection?**

3. **What is the recommended course of treatment?**

Case Study Answers

CASE STUDY 1

1. The appendix (as well as tonsils and Peyer's patches) is a representative lymphoid tissue found in and around mucosal epithelia (referred to as MALT, or mucosa-associated lymphoid tissue). Within the appendix, specialized resident intraepithelial lymphocytes with potent cytolytic and immunoregulatory capacities monitor mucosal tissue to help defend against pathogenic infection.

2. Obstruction of the appendix lumen is the primary cause of appendicitis, leading to tissue distention from excessive accumulated intraluminal fluid. The most common cause of luminal obstruction is lymphoid follicle hyperplasia, at times reflective of high bacterial burden and overaggressive immune response. Ineffective lymphatic drainage allows bacterial invasion within the appendix wall, with high polymorphonuclear cell reactivity and resultant inflammation.

3. Standard therapy involves removal of the inflamed appendix through a procedure aptly named appendectomy; serious complications may result if the appendix ruptures. A ruptured appendix can lead to peritonitis from leakage of trapped bacteria into the abdomen. Often, abscess formation will occur, comprising a swollen mass filled with fluid and bacteria and pus (dead and dying neutrophils trying to control spread of infection). Peritoneal bacteria often release endotoxins, such as lipopolysaccharides (LPSs), contributing to septic events and the possibility of secondary organ failure.

CASE STUDY 2

1. The deficiency is a compromise of both the reticuloendothelial (RES) system and adaptive immunity due to the congenital absence of a spleen. The major shortcoming is a loss of mononuclear phagocytes to clear pathogenic organisms from the blood. Secondarily, there is a loss of B- and T-cell mass, which ultimately may be largely compensated at the level of systemic lymphoid tissue. The individual is predisposed to morbidity and mortality from encapsulated organisms such as *Streptococcus pneumoniae*, *Haemophilus influenzae*, and *Neisseria meningitides* (meningococcus), which require antibody response for protection.

2. Loss of a spleen would be more detrimental to a child than to an adult primarily because of a previously established immune response (B cells and their ability to produce specific antibodies) to bacterial antigens in the adult. In the adult, preexisting memory B cells surviving in other tissues (e.g., lymph nodes, GALT, MALT, and BALT) may be activated, although the overall response in these adults typically is diminished. In the child, there is less likely to be a preexisting memory population. The lack of splenic lymphoid tissue to process antigen greatly decreases the opportunity for B-cell activation and further production of plasma cells and memory B cells. Additional concerns include lowered specific immunoglobulin production, and decreased complement fixation associated with the classical component pathway.

3. Medical care involves antibiotic prophylaxis, immunizations, aggressive management of the suspected infection, and parent education. Antibiotic prophylaxis is initiated immediately upon the diagnosis because patients are considered immunocompromised. Patients should receive standard immunizations, especially conjugated *H. influenzae* type b and pneumococcal vaccines. Asplenic patients are at an increased risk for sepsis, especially from gram-positive organisms. Parents must be educated to remain vigilant to detect symptoms of infection, so that early detection will allow aggressive management.

CASE STUDY 3

1. Multiple myeloma (also called plasma cell myeloma) is a progressive cancer of the plasma cell, a mature B cell that functionally produces immunoglobulins. Multiple myeloma is characterized by excessive numbers of abnormal clonal plasma cells in the bone marrow and overproduction of intact monoclonal immunoglobulin (of any isotype) or Bence-Jones protein (circulating monoclonal κ and λ light chains in the absence of heavy chains). Because the

myeloma cells are identical, they all produce the same immunoglobulin protein, called monoclonal (M) protein, in large quantities.

2. Transformation of a B cell to a malignant plasma cell involves processes that generate genetic abnormalities, sometimes including translocation of chromosomes near the heavy chain locus. The outcome is the allowance of malignant cells to divide unchecked. Myeloma cells that invade bone can establish masses, or plasmacytomas, that produce growth factors and vascular endothelial growth factor (VEGF) to promote angiogenesis. Eventually multiple small lesions form and spread into large bone cavities throughout the body, giving rise to anemia and reduced polymorphonuclear cell production owing to displacement of functional hematopoietic stem cells.

3. Although high levels of circulating antibody exist, the antibodies produced are monoclonal in nature. The hypergammaglobulinemia comes at the relative expense of normal immunoglobulin production. In essence, the patient becomes functionally antibody deficient in spite of high numbers of nonspecific antibodies in circulation. This, combined with anemic and neutropenic conditions, raises susceptibility to pyogenic bacteria requiring specific antibody response for clearance of infectious organisms.

CASE STUDY 4

1. DiGeorge syndrome is a rare form of primary immunodeficiency, the basis for which is congenital absence or aplasia of the thymus due to defects during embryogenesis stemming from a large deletion from chromosome 22.

2. T lymphocytes released from the bone marrow migrate to the thymus, where further development and education into functional phenotypes occur. Thymic education includes removal of self-reactive T lymphocytes and commitment of remaining cells to helper (CD4$^+$) or cytotoxic (CD8$^+$) phenotypes. In the absence of a thymus, maturation of T lymphocytes does not occur, and CD3$^+$, CD4$^+$, and CD8$^+$ populations are particularly low.

3. The prognosis is dependent upon the severity of T lymphocyte compromise. Opportunistic infections occurring because of severe immunodeficiency are the second most common cause of death in patients with Di George syndrome. Although B lymphocytes are present and serum IgG levels are typically normal, the functionality of the B-cell response is limited owing to lack of help from antigen-specific T$_H$. Common infections manifest as ear and sinus infections, pneumonia, infectious diarrhea, and severe thrush (*Candida*). Antibiotic treatment assists in the short term, but long-term therapeutic intervention dictates strengthening the immune system by bone marrow transplantation and possibly thymus transplantation to recover maturation of the T-cell response.

CASE STUDY 5

1. It is common for individuals to be maintained on immunosuppressive agents for long periods following major organ transplantation. The symptoms described in this patient overlap with early stages of graft rejection; however, in this case the cause was viral. Immunosuppression is the critical postoperative factor that predisposes to infection in transplant recipients, as agents dampen immune function; patients typically remain on low levels of therapeutics for the rest of their lives. Dampening of T$_H$ and T cytotoxic lymphocytic responses specifically limits the ability to fight against viral infection, thus contributing to the disease state in this person.

2. The human leukocyte antigens (HLA) are a complex set of molecules expressed on the surface of cells. These molecules, also referred to as major histocompatibility complex molecules (MHC), are product s of polymorphic genes that are the principal determinants of whether an organ is deemed as self or nonself. These molecules present antigen to T lymphocytes as a method of regulating immune response. In general, class I MHC molecules present peptides derived from endogenous pathways to cytotoxic lymphocytes, while class II MHC molecules present exogenous antigens to T$_H$ lymphocytes. Donor tissue must match closely in HLA alleles for acceptance by the recipient.

3. In addition to parainfluenza virus, other community-based respiratory viruses are commonly found in immunosuppressed transplant patients, including influenza, respiratory syncytial virus (RSV), herpesvirus, varicella virus, and adenovirus. Furthermore, cytomegalovirus (CMV) is quite common, most likely related to the patient's prior CMV status (upwards of 80% of the adult population have been exposed to CMV).

CASE STUDY 6

1. LAD is an autosomal recessive disorder in which there is a failure to express surface integrins on myeloid and lymphoid cells. Migration of activated polymorphonuclear cells and lymphocytes to sites of inflammation require expression of selectins on endothelial cells and concurrent binding by ligands on rolling leukocytes. Directed diapedesis ensues through integrin interactions (via CD18, a surface β_2-integrin). Lack of CD18 results in inefficient entry of circulating leukocytes to sites of inflammation. Additionally, CD18 serves as a complement receptor on myeloid cells (for C3b), assisting with phagocytosis and efficient microbicidal activity in neutrophil, monocyte, and macrophage populations.

2. The NBT test allows examination of bactericidal activity of polymorphonuclear cells. NBT is an electron acceptor that

is reduced in the presence of free O_2 radicals to form a blue compound, formazan. NBT is added to activated white blood cells. Neutrophils produce reactive oxygen species (ROS) when stimulated, a function that assists in bactericidal activity. The ROS produced also turns NBT from a clear color to a deep blue. In this patient, there is no deficiency in production of ROS; rather, additional assays of random migration and chemotaxis were necessary to define phenotypic deficiencies.

3. Most patients with LAD have a poor outcome, with few infants surviving past 1 year of age. Bacterial infections and severe viral infections are responsible for most deaths. The most common bacterial agents are the *Staphylococcus* species and enteric gram-negative bacteria. Infection with fungal agents (such as *Candida albicans*) are also common. In many cases, bone marrow and other stem cell transplantation procedures have proved effective at prolonging survival.

CASE STUDY 7

1. Omenn's syndrome is an autosomal recessive form of severe combined immunodeficiency (SCID) characterized by susceptibility to fungal, bacterial, and viral infections. The molecular defect is linked to defects in either of the recombinase-activating genes, *RAG-1* or *RAG-2*, which control generation of antigen-binding diversity by assembly of the genes encoding variable (V), diversity (D), and joining (J) domains for both the T-cell receptor (TCR) and the B-cell receptor (antibody). The inability to productively rearrange exons required for T- and B-cell receptors leads to poorly functional T cells and absent B cells.

2. The remaining *RAG* gene remains functional, albeit deficient in complete maturation of lymphocytes without the other gene. It is hypothesized that a subpopulation of T_H lymphocytes of the T_H2 variety are expanded, possibly as a result of increased exposure to inadequately cleared antigens and resulting expansion of a minor oligoclonal population of activated and antigen-stimulated cells. These T_H2 produce elevated levels of interleukin 4 (IL-4) and interleukin 5 (IL-5), cytokines that mediate eosinophilia. Of interest, high production of nonspecific IgE (hyperimmunoglobulinemia E) may also occur in these patients. Likewise, the limited repertoire of productive lymphocytes is likely to show decreased responses to specific antigens and variable responses to nonspecific mitogens.

3. Mortality and morbidity levels are increased in all SCID patients, regardless of the specific molecular defect. Life-threatening viral, bacterial, and fungal infections are prominent in Omenn's syndrome patients, as in other types of SCID. A higher incidence of malignancies occurs, most likely due to loss of regulating cytotoxic

lymphocytes. Prophylactic antibiotics are warranted. Bone marrow transplantation is usually successful to reconstitute immune surveillance; however, care should be taken to avoid the common complication of chronic graft-versus-host disease (GVHD).

CASE STUDY 8

1. Multiple sclerosis is a disease of the central nervous system affecting the nerves of the brain and spinal cord. Myelin, produced in the brain and spinal cord by oligodendrocytes, forms a protective coat around axons, allowing nondisruption of electric impulses away from nerve cells. It is thought that immunoreactive T lymphocytes contribute to destruction of the myelin sheath, recognizing self-tissue as foreign. This in turn assists in the production of autoantibodies from self-reactive B lymphocytes. Ultimately, this leads to disease manifestation.

2. The process involves destruction of myelin (demyelination), producing multiple patches of hard, scarred tissue called plaques; "sclerosis" (Greek) means hard. Sodium ion channels, which boost electrical charges between nerves, are clustered at the nodes of Ranvier. These channels are disrupted, leading to interruption of signal transmission between cells within the nervous system when sodium ions are not able to boost impulses.

3. It is not clear why some autoimmune events occur in everyone, yet not everyone develops autoimmune disease. Genetic factors certainly play a role in development of MS, with risk factors higher in first-degree relatives and identical twins. However, no single gene has been identified to trigger autoimmune conditions. Rather, a combination of genetic factors most likely renders individuals more susceptible to disease manifestation. It is also likely that environmental factors can trigger the autoimmune response, be it chemical or infectious in nature. Although certain infections are suspected to trigger autoimmune MS (e.g., herpesviruses), no single agent to date has been identified. Although they are not causative, both trauma and stress can exacerbate disease symptoms.

CASE STUDY 9

1. Acute myelogenous leukemia is a type of blood cancer in which myeloid cells become cancerous, usually due to damage of DNA within developing cells of the bone marrow. The resulting damage causes chromosomal abnormalities that disrupt genes encoding for transcription required for stem cell differentiation into specific blood phenotypes.

2. Bone marrow transplantation (also referred to as stem cell transplantation) is an excellent clinical tool to reconstitute normal immune and hematopoietic function in patients undergoing cancer chemotherapy. The major complications include increased susceptibility to infection from opportunistic organisms or latent viral entities due to lack of mature lymphocytes specific to ward off infecting agents. As new cells are generated in the host, the ability to fight infection remanifests. Another potential adverse effect can occur when the source of bone marrow used for transplantation is allogeneic (not syngeneic), leading to graft-versus-host disease (GVHD) over time. The basis of GVHD is that mature donor lymphocytes transferred to the recipient may show reactivity to mismatched antigens (major histocompatibility antigens or ABO groups) residing on recipient tissue. In all cases, laboratory tissue typing and mixed lymphocyte reactions (culturing donor and recipient cells together) would be performed to ascertain reactivity between new and existing cell populations.

3. The ABO blood groups are carbohydrate moieties present on erythrocytes that represent important antigens to be accounted for to ensure safe blood transfusions. Individuals naturally develop antibodies (called isoantibodies) specific for ABO antigens that they do not express. If the individual receives a transfusion of blood containing incompatible ABO antigens, isoantibodies will cause agglutination of the donor cells, called isohemagglutination.

4. The patient had undergone ablation of precursor stem cells, thus limiting his reactivity to the foreign donor cells. However, persistent peripheral cells within the host may have survived with enough reactivity to attack new donor cells; immunosuppressive agents were administered to allow the new donor stem cells to inhabit the bone marrow and limit destruction prior to successful reconstitution of host immune function.

CASE STUDY 10

1. Toxic shock syndrome (TSS) is a severe illness associated with *Staphylococcus aureus* infection, characterized by fever, nausea, diffuse erythema, and shock. It typically occurs in menstruating females using tampons, primarily when saturated tampons are not changed often, allowing unchecked growth of microorganisms. However, TSS is not limited to women and may occur in any individual exposed to large numbers of *S. aureus*.

2. The superantigens staphylococcal enterotoxin and toxin-1 are responsible for toxic shock syndrome. Superantigens are defined by their ability to stimulate a large fraction of T cells via interaction with the T-cell receptor (TCR), usually through the variable beta (Vβ) domain. In this manner, the superantigen circumvents normal processing and directly links the TCR with the major histocompatibility (MHC)

class II molecule, causing cells to differentiate into effector cells that release high levels of cytokines. Because the number of T cells that share Vβ domains is high (up to 10% of all T cells), large numbers of T cells (regardless of antigen specificity) may be activated by superantigens, causing massive release of cytokines and subsequent symptoms of shock and host injury.

3. The overwhelming number of cytokines released from activated T cells caused a cascade of effects at both local and systemic levels. Cytokines released include IL-2, TNF-α, and IL-1β. IL-2 is a mitogenic stimulatory factor for T cells, thus furthering the cascade of T-cell activity. Both TNF-α and IL-1β cause activation of vascular endothelium and increased vascular permeability, thus contributing to hypotensive shock in the patient as fluid accumulation in vascular beds occurred. Local responses also included direct tissue damage, since TNF-α can be a necrotic factor at high concentrations. These same cytokines, along with IL-6, evoke systemic effects including fever production, mobilization of shock-related metabolites, and induction of acute-phase protein production. This was manifested by elevated enzyme levels, which were further indicative of destruction of renal and hepatic tissue.

CASE STUDY 11

1. The finding of boxcar-shaped, gram-positive rods that do not grow aerobically is consistent with *Clostridium perfringens*, frequently associated with gas gangrene (see Chapter 12). Spores of the organism persist in soil; introduction of organisms into wound areas followed by toxin production destroys skin and muscle tissue. The bacteria grow and manufacture "gas" as a by-product, often detectable by radiographs or scans of the wounded area. *C. perfringens* is also the causative agent for more common disease-associated food poisoning due to gut-released enterotoxins.

2. *Clostridium* spp produce virulence factors, including a lecithinase that is capable of lysing polymorphonuclear cells, thus the lack of cellularity in the tissue biopsy. The α-toxin lecithinase (a phospholipase C) plays a central role in development of gas gangrene pathogenesis, while limiting the innate immune system response. Additional tissue-destructive factors released include a protease, hyaluronidase, collagenase, and general hemolysins.

3. If infection is not treated immediately and aggressively, mortality rates are above 40%. Aggressive penicillin antibiotic therapy is warranted with accompanying surgical débridement. If the infection does not respond to this therapy, then amputation above the affected area is warranted to limit spread through draining lymphatics. Because the organism is anaerobic, hyperbaric chamber treatment (O_2-rich atmosphere) is useful.

CASE STUDY 12

1. Organisms engulfed by macrophages stimulate responses leading to exudative (pneumonia-like) or granulomatous lesions. The granulomatous lesions are characterized by giant multinucleated cells that are surrounded by lymphocytes, forming the basis of a tubercle. Immunologic responses to the persisting organism trigger destructive pathology and necrotic events, leaving a caseous center to the granuloma. Eventual erosion of lesions into bronchial airways leads to spread of disease.

2. Risk factors such as smoking habits, alcohol consumption, family history of tuberculosis, and lifetime work history all contribute to potential for disease. A social worker would have greater exposure to mycobacteria from indigent populations with limited access to health care. In this patient, smoking for many years most likely impaired native lung macrophage function, contributing to the progression from infection to manifestation of disease. Other factors, such as age and ethnic origin, are also associated with an increased risk of infection progressing to disease.

3. Because of the slow growth doubling of mycobacteria (18–24 hours), therapeutic intervention is made over a lengthy period. The Centers for Disease Control and Prevention (CDC) recommends multidrug treatment with isoniazid, rifampin, pyrazinamide, and ethambutol or streptomycin for tuberculosis for compliant patients with fully susceptible organisms. These drugs are taken daily for 2 months followed by daily isoniazid and rifampin therapy for an additional 4 months. Directly observed therapy (DOT) is strongly considered in all patients to limit development of multidrug-resistant organisms in uncompliant patients. Preventative measures in immunocompromised individuals are more aggressive.

4. The acid-fast smear plays an important diagnostic role in mycobacterial infections. The ability to retain aryl methane dyes (carbolfuchsin and auramine O) within the lipid-rich mycobacterial cell wall, after washing with alcohol or weak acids, is a primary feature of mycobacteria. Both Ziehl-Neelsen and Kinyoun methods take advantage of this property to allow quick identification of slowly growing organisms in sputum samples.

CASE STUDY 13

1. Sexual transmission is the primary mode for the spread of HSV-2, and it is likely that the patient had a encounter with an infected individual many years ago. At that time, symptoms were most likely limited to herpetic lesions of the genital area. In general, herpesviruses start off with acute infection but progress to lifelong latent infection with periodic reactivation of symptomatic infection.

2. HSV-2 is known for its neurovirulent properties, with latency established in nerve root ganglia. Aseptic meningitis is the main neurologic complication of reactivation of HSV-2 infection. Although herpes-induced encephalitis may occur, it is relatively rare. Rather, herpes-related meningitis occurs in a low but significant number of cases, stemming from primary genital HSV-2. The meningitis is self-limited (lasting less than a week) with only rare persisting neurologic impairment. HSV-2 may also cause benign recurrent lymphocytic meningitis, with lingering presence of elevated activated immune cells and occasional presence of Mollaret cells (giant epithelioid cells of mononuclear origin) in cerebrospinal fluid. Neuralgias are also associated with reactivation infection.

3. Latent HSV can be reactivated by fever, trauma, emotional stress, excessive sunlight, and even menstruation in females. Notably, reactivation is more frequent and severe in immunocompromised patients owing to lack of T_H cell and cytotoxic cell control during early reactivation events. Systemic viral diseases may also trigger general gastroenteritis, possibly due to cytokine cascades released during aggressive T-cell responses.

CASE STUDY 14

1. Because the patient is immunocompromised with low CD4+ cell numbers, it is likely that an opportunistic infection is the causative agent for the gastrointestinal pathology. Some of the more common agents include *Cryptosporidium*, *Histoplasma*, *Entamoeba histolytica* (amebiasis), and *Campylobacter* spp. In addition, complications due to disseminated *Mycobacteria* cannot be ruled out; a negative PPD test may indicate loss of $CD4^+$ cell function rather than lack of exposure.

2. Treatment depends upon identification of the opportunistic infection. Because of the high likelihood of a fungal agent, administration of intravenous amphotericin B is warranted, followed by maintenance therapy with oral itraconazole or fluconazole. For *Cryptosporidium*, paromomycin and azithromycin are recommended. For general bacterial infections in the lower intestine, clarithromycin and amoxicillin are first choices unless a drug-resistant strain is detected. In all cases, improvement of the immune system and decrease in human immunodeficiency virus (HIV) viral loads (through use of antiviral therapy) will lead to long-lasting results.

3. HAART is an acronym for highly active antiretroviral therapy, and it represents guidelines established to reduce HIV viral burdens to ultimately limit the occurrence of opportunistic infections in immunocompromised individuals. A complex mixture of antiretroviral drugs are used that act at different stages of the HIV life cycle. These drugs include reverse transcriptase inhibitors (both nucleoside and non-nucleoside inhibitors),

nucleotide analog reverse transcriptase inhibitors, protease inhibitors, and cell fusion inhibitors, which limit entry of virus into cells.

CASE STUDY 15

1. Prematurity and surgery are the primary predisposing risk factors for candidiasis. Neonates with weakened immune function or defects in mounting a cellular immune response show decreased resistance to fungal infections. Likewise, patients with defects in neutrophil function are also at risk for disseminated disease.

2. Nosocomial acquisition is the most likely form of transmission as a result of contamination of the disposable vascular device (the percutaneously inserted central line). The point of entry for the organism would be the catheter; vascular lines should be monitored to ensure cleanliness to limit infections. Neonatal candidiasis may also occur by vertical transmission (from mother to child during birth), although symptoms would most likely have been manifested earlier in this case.

3. Current therapeutic treatment involves rapid intravenous administration of amphotericin B (or another antifungal agent). If candidemia is not treated immediately, its potential to cause extensive tissue invasion is increased, possibly leading to osteomyelitis, endocarditis, or meningitis. Invasive candidemia may also affect bones and joints and kidney tissue, leading to renal insufficiency. In the majority of cases, catheter-related candidemia will resolve soon after catheter removal and initiation of therapy.

CASE STUDY 16

1. Differential diagnoses include infectious and neoplastic diseases of the liver and gallbladder disease (hence the yellowish sclera). Specific etiologies are hepatocellular cancer or intestinal/hepatic parasitic infection (e.g., *Schistosoma mansoni* or *Strongyloides stercoralis*). Esophagogastroduodenoscopic biopsy should be performed. In this case, histologic examination of collected tissue revealed intense infiltrate of polymorphonuclear leukocytes, with a predominance of eosinophils. *S. stercoralis* was positively identified.

2. Although *S. stercoralis* is an intestinal nematode, larvae occasionally spread to the respiratory tract, resulting in clinical symptoms ranging from cough to hemoptysis and pulmonary infiltrates. The filariform larvae of *S. stercoralis* may also be encountered in respiratory specimens but are more commonly seen in superinfection in immunosuppressed individuals.

3. *Strongyloides* may be treated with albendazole or thiabendazole. However, it should be noted that anthelmintic therapy works poorly against larvae; treatment must therefore wait for established infection. If *S. stercoralis* is diagnosed in early stages (during larval migration to lung tissue), symptomatic treatment with inhaled beta-agonists is sufficient; corticosteroid therapy is not recommended, since it leads to compromise of cell-mediated immunity, allowing massive proliferation and widespread dissemination of larvae.

Index

Note: Page numbers followed by f indicate figures; those followed by t indicate tables; and those followed by b indicate boxed material.